Exceptional Aging:
Fierce Food &
Smart Supplements

The nutrition formula for vitality after 50

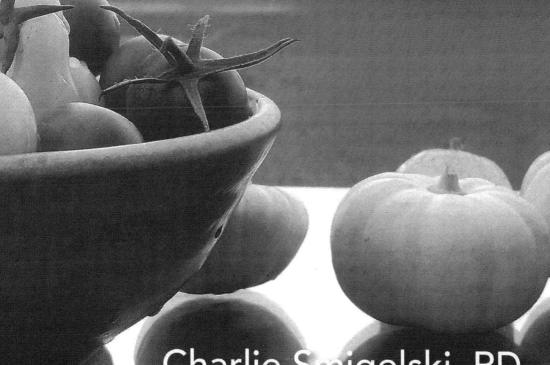

Charlie Smigelski, RD

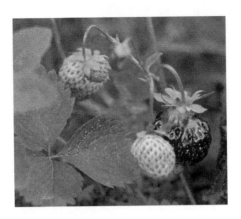

**Special thanks to Jeff, Amy, Ken and Roz for editing help
and to all who supported me in this effort.**

A special note of appreciation to my patients who took the risk and trusted my advice and improved their health. They are a big part of my nourishment.

ISBN: 978–0–692–17852–2

Book design, photography & illustrations by Jeffry Pike, jeffry@pikecreates.com.

Printed by Charlie Smigelski, in the United States of America.
First printing edition 2018.

charlie@charliesmigelskird.com
https://charlienutrition.com/

Preamble
Nutrition To Keep You At Your Best

Nutrition is about repairing you. After age 50, when you are smarter/better informed about eating, you can change old concepts of vitality in later years. While eating a great diet provides a crucial foundation, recent nutrition studies prove that you can feel even stronger and fitter when you know about some key supplements that the body needs in greater quantity after age 50.

Waking up today, on the trek from bedroom to kitchen, did you move comfortably, painlessly, energetically? Last night's supper and evening snacks were supposed to restore your body while you slept, like repairing legs from yesterday's "brisk walk" that your doctor prescribed for you. So, how did you do? Are you feeling fit today? Maybe you're sluggish because the magnesium or B-vitamins weren't there at 4 am when the protein assembly line needed a catalytic nudge to link some amino acids to muscle fibers? At the end of the workday, are your ankles a little puffy? Is fluid pooling there at the far end of your body because your heart just doesn't have enough oomph to pump the liquids against gravity, from your feet, back up through your calves and thighs? It is the simple truth: the groceries you buy, the meals and snacks you eat, the vitamins you take; these are what keep your muscle, bone, brain and immune cells operating at their best. Your nutrition choices, past and present, decide the performance quality of your cells, and after age 50 they matter even more.

Your doctor often suggests medicines when you have complaints. Take one pill to reduce blood pressure; take a different pill to stop the pain of arthritis. The drugs stop the hurt; but don't help the underlying problem: the failure of the joint cells to heal. Remember, you are not suffering from an ibuprofen deficiency; you have an "itis," an inflammation, because cells are not mending well enough. As many of you know, the drugs have their own set of complications, and usually some undesirable side effects. At this point in life, you want to focus on having all systems at their metabolic best, otherwise the stack of pills for managing symptoms will continue to mount. This book details the foods you could eat, plus the vitamins and other supplements you can take, for fitness and cell rejuvenation. Doing what this book suggests could likely reduce your need for medicines.

This book is about smart food and nutrition choices. Don't let the advice lapse into feeling like yet another set of food rules to live by. View it, instead, as ideas to move you into a stronger place. Food is still supposed to be fun. It can have tremendous spiritual and psychological power too. We're pretty grumpy characters if we're deprived of it for many hours or days. In fact, we are hot-wired to needing food, ranking it more important than shelter and companionship in our basic instinctive needs.[1] Food brightens our mood too: succulent strawberries and luscious whip cream on a crispy sweet biscuit perk up a summer supper, for sure. OK, eat up.

Part 1 of this book provides the basic info for being fierce with food.

Part 2 gives you basic science information about aging, and how nutrients impact that physiology.

Part 3 helps you create a detailed eating plan for yourself.

Part 4 will make you very smart about how a number of nutrition supplements will help your body function better, and do it safely.

Part 5 is a head to toe review of ailments that you can mend with fierce foods and smart supplements.

Part 6 provides special details on carbohydrate processing (diabetes too) and immune function: two areas of particular importance as people age.

Part 7 introduces you to an energy healing treatment that can make your nutrition therapies even more dynamic.

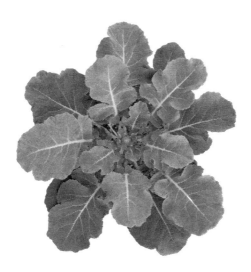

Table of Contents

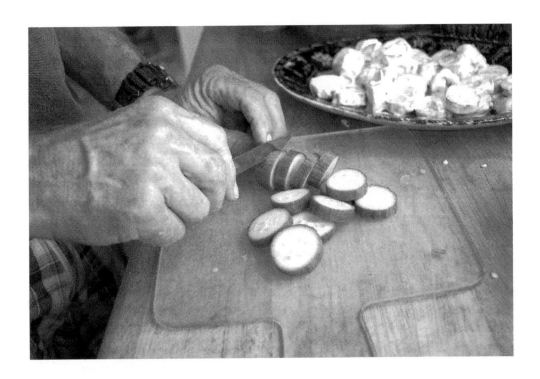

Best Nutrition
Three Fundamental Concepts

**For your body to function at its best,
have the food you eat supply the materials that
your caveperson-era genes are expecting.**

Here is a core idea, a fundamental concept to utilize in making the most of your food choices. Have the food you eat be food that your caveman or cavewoman genes are expecting to receive, to do the work of replenishing your system today. We carry the gene product of about 100,000 years of evolution as *homo sapiens*.[2]

**Will the food you are about to eat hinder the repair systems and
aggravate the operating cells of your body?**

There is also the opposite concept: when thinking about what to eat, ask whether this food will irritate your cellular systems, and be more of a burden on repair activities? The idea is not to make a health food freak of you, but a lot of what passes for routine cuisine these days is either lacking in key repair materials, or providing elements that are annoying or mildly toxic to the body.

**Have the food you eat be nourishing to your cells,
but also to the psychological and spiritual you.**

One more perspective, as you pull breakfast or lunch together, what are you really nourishing? There is the physical part of you that may be about to go out and pedal a bicycle for an hour or two, or go sit through a ninety-minute committee meeting. Both activities require steady fuel and energy. A smart blend of fats, carbohydrates and protein will sustain you.

To stay focused on eating well for the long haul, it also helps to have a philosophical component to your food selection process. Do you actually look forward to breakfast, or lunch? Why, or why not? Could you imagine food as fun: the tropical aroma of a mango, or the summer sweetness of blueberries, to start your day off on a good note? Will lunch today, turkey on whole wheat, with lettuce, tomato, and mustard, be the same as it has been for the past 34 days? If lunch were a little more exciting, what would that do for your wellbeing today? Would "cowboy caviar": black beans, corn, diced tomato, onion plus green pepper, along with some maple-smoked chicken sausage, feel just a little livelier? Is it that much extra work to make the salad at home and bring it to the office, or would just some planning ahead make it happen? Maybe you start with gourmet Thursdays, just to perk up the latter part of the workweek? This meal can nourish your arms and legs, but also feed brain cells for the next few hours.

Assembling a Really Good Diet for Yourself

As you think about eating well, think about assembling your daily diet in a series of steps.

1. **Figure out proteins, and have them at all three meals:** breakfast, lunch, and dinner. These are foods for structure. As we age, research is showing that we need more protein, not less.[3]

2. **Plan on eating a lot of vegetables at both lunch and dinner.** You need more vegetables than you think, and you likely can't meet all your needs by having them just at supper.[4][5]

3. **Stock up on fruits.** You want to eat them 3 to 4 times a day. Remember 7 days a week, times 3 per day … do you have 21 fruit items in your grocery cart this week?

4. **Nuts and seeds contain crucial oils that form cell membranes and brain cell structure.** A good idea is to consume a handful of nuts and of seeds every day.

5. **Pick starches (carbohydrates) as the remaining part of your fuel source.** Select wisely; you need carbohydrates for fuel but think about portions. In aging, the hormone insulin makes over-sized servings of starches turn to fat faster.[6]

PART 1:

All The Food Details: Groceries and Meals

The next dozen or so pages of this book discuss food groups and individual items within the categories. Read them so that you can learn about particularly good elements in certain foods. You might find foods you already like, and that are actually especially good for you.

This section has sample menus for the day. Some recipes will be sprinkled thoughout the book, so you can enjoy some new foods in a tasty way.

*The way to think about choosing proteins,
and many other good foods, is to think back to
selections that reflect caveman era choices.*

Protein
Providing Amino Acids that Nourish Body and Brain

Your body is expecting you to crawl out of your hut or cave this morning, go over
to the river, lake or ocean, smack a fish over the head, or grab some clams, and start
dining. Maybe you'll sneak up on a bird, grab it and eat it. One important concept
here: having protein for breakfast is a critical part of your good nutrition plan.

Your body is in a constant state of renewal. The body assembles amino acids
into protein units, such as muscles and immune cells. Dietary protein is your
best source of amino acids. You are making new liver, intestine and skin cells
every day. You are also making millions of immune cells to fight off the viruses or
germs you get from living in the modern world.

To support the repair efforts in all these body parts, eat good protein foods,
and enough of them.

Protein needs rise as we age. Especially focus on repairing muscles, not just
bones. Bone loss — osteoporosis — gets a lot of publicity because pharmaceutical
companies advertise treatment drugs,[7] but subtle loss of muscle is a far more
common and serious clinical issue. It is a lack of muscle strength that causes older
people to fall, and then break a hip. Weak bones are not what provoke falls. Loss
of muscle, known as "sarcopenia" is a bigger problem than people and doctors
appreciate. In a 2002 Connecticut study, 20% of people over 64 showed signifcant
muscle loss, and over age 80, 30% had significant losses.[8]

So let's talk smart protein choices. Eggs are a very good choice: even better
when they are "omega-3 eggs". These are eggs produced by chickens that were
fed more greens, so they contain better quality fats in their yolks. Egg yolks have
many brain-nourishing compounds too. As the main protein source at a meal,
one egg is not enough; eat two. Fish and seafood are always good sources of
protein. Fish with omega-3 fats is extra good. Just so you know, tuna does not
have much omega-3. Have wild Alaskan salmon instead (see recipe on page 40).
You may have been told that shrimp or other shellfish have a lot of cholesterol, so
avoid them: not true. These contain plant sterols, but not excessive cholesterol.
Shrimp with cocktail sauce: perfect. Shrimp or scallops seared in a pan with a
little olive oil and garlic: excellent.

Protein concepts and sources

Protein concepts

When you think about eating to repair your body, you want to think about eating proteins from the streams, lakes and oceans, or low fat land items.

- The more you eat from the lefthand column of the list below the better off you are.
- The fish in **bold type** have more "omega-3 oils", which have natural anti-inflammatory properties. Other fish are still great choices, because they are low fat and have minimal saturated fat.
- You want to eat protein at breakfast, lunch, and dinner.
- Whey protein is a great repair protein. Blend it with fruit for smoothies at breakfast.

Sources

Protein source in **bold type** are extra fierce.

Blue fish	**Whey protein powder**	Pork tenderloin
Cod	No fat/Low fat cottage	Lite/Low fat cheeses
Flounder	cheese	Omega-3 eggs
Haddock	Egg whites/EggBeaters	
Herring	Veggie burger	***Grass-fed is best:***
Lobster	Turkey breast	Lamb chops
Salmon	Turkey ham	Lean beef
Sardines	Turkey sausage	Cheese, *especially*
Shrimp	Chicken breast	goat & sheep
Scallops	Chicken legs	
Trout	Chicken thighs	Collagen peptides
Tuna	Pork chop	

Chicken, turkey, lamb, pork and cow are also good sources of protein. In this era of industrial-strength food production, though, eating grass-fed and organic is an important concept if you can afford the extra cost. Feedlot raised, grain-fed modern cows and pigs sometimes contain fats that the body is not accustomed to dealing with. Antibiotic residue may also be likely.

In ancient times, hunters and gatherers chased down deer or wild boar, but the flesh of wild animals is very lean when they grow in their natural state. The wild animals ate wild grasses, meaning their flesh contained omega-3 fats. Whenever you can, buy products that are "grass-fed" and "antibiotic-free." You have less worries about eating "red meat" then. Enjoy without guilt!

Cheese is another whole story. In the famous Mediterranean Diet, in its purest form on the island of Crete, the cheese and ice cream have omega-3 fats, because all the dairy-producing animals were grass-fed. Much of the dairy tends to come from goat and sheep milk, as another point of interest.[9] In the US, the saturated fat from factory farm dairy is missing some good elements, like vitamin K2, and conjugated linoleic acid (CLA). So stick to lower fat dairy items when you can. Buy grass-fed organic when you want to enjoy full fat cheese, and look for goat and sheep cheeses.

In hunting and gathering times, people did meet about half their protein needs with plant-origin amino acids. Many came from leaves, shoots and vegetables. In the Mediterranean Diet, legumes also provide a decent amount of protein. For people choosing to be vegetarian, I would still encourage modest doses of dairy or eggs to support getting adequate amounts of protein to meet the needs of an aging person. For vegans, you need to pay attention to getting some supplemental protein servings from items like soy and pea powders.

Remember the simple idea: your body expects much of your protein to come from the ocean, or streams and rivers, plus some from land as plants or eggs. Proteins with too much saturated fat change the physical and metabolic performance of your cells. Don't add the hassle of coping with too much modern thick grease to the work of self-repair. Limit the added burden of eating conventional steaks, burgers, and full fat cheese to a few events per week.

Vegetables
Restocking Your Cells with Minerals

Another caveman diet idea: in the olden days, people got huge amounts of nutrition from vegetables. They wandered around munching leaves and shoots like Swiss chard, collards, and asparagus all day. Imagine eating 5 or 7 bags of leaves, I mean large bowls of salad, in a day. You probably aren't doing this now, but in a sense, it is what your body is expecting, is certainly ready for, and likes to receive.

Vegetables are a major source of crucial minerals. Minerals are structural material for you, like the calcium in bones. Minerals also nudge along important chemical reactions. Examples are iron helping red blood cell hemoglobin carry

Here's the word on vegetables

Vegetable concepts

Here is a list of 30 vegetables to remind you of the many choices you have. In this list, the vegetables in the **bold type** (below) are the ones with the most vitamins or minerals or both.

- Eat at least a cup of vegetables at both lunch and supper. Snacking on vegetables is also good, too.

- You might be someone who is just not into eating vegetables. At least try to have one cup of a vegetable in bold face below. Then eat an extra piece of fruit each day, to make up for the fiber you are missing.

- While fresh and frozen are the best, even canned vegetables still offer some minerals and fiber.

- The gooey fiber in okra and eggplant is especially good for lowering cholesterol.

- Ever tried Swiss chard? It's a super-food with a serious magnesium content.

Sources

Vegetables in **bold type** have more vitamins or minerals or both.

Asparagus	Dark green lettuce	Pea pods
Bok choy	Eggplant	**Purslane**
Broccoli	Green/yellow beans	**Spinach**
Brussels sprouts	Green/red/hot peppers	Summer squash
Cabbage	Kale	**Swiss chard**
Carrots	**Mushrooms**	**Tomatoes**
Cauliflower	**Mustard greens**	Tomato sauce
Celery	**Okra**	**Winter squash**
Collard greens	Onion	Zucchini squash
Cucumbers	**Parsley**	
Dandelion Greens	Parsnip	

oxygen, or magnesium helping calcium stay in bones, and magnesium helping muscles relax.

Eating many minerals, like potassium, magnesium, selenium and zinc is the key to optimum operation of all kinds of hormones and repair enzymes. Blood pressure stays lower, insulin manages blood sugar better, and bones rebuild stronger, all thanks to small, but crucial, amounts of minerals in vegetables.

You often hear about the Mediterranean Diet which is based on the food intake of people on the island of Crete. People there seem to consume 245 kilograms of vegetables and fruits per year. Compared this to the 150 kg in Italy and France, and 90 kg in Finland.[10] Do some math:

Convert kilograms to pounds $\longrightarrow$ 245 kg x 2.2 lbs = ~540 lbs/yr.
Daily intake of plant material $\longrightarrow$ 540 lbs / 365 days = 1.5 lbs/day

So, don't be patting yourself on the back because you ate a splash of lettuce and tomato on your sandwich at lunch. When you have 2 quarts of salad, or 3 huge carrots, or 2 tomatoes, a whole green pepper plus a few mushrooms at lunch, then you get to feel proud.

There is always room for improvement in eating vegetables. The cafeteria at work may not have a great selection, but do what you can. If the vegetables are kind of soft and tired, toss them in some soup to make them taste a little better.

At the salad bar, what vegetables look good today? The lettuce looks limp, so maybe your salad is just celery and mushrooms: fine; those two foods are very good blood pressure therapy. Eat a cereal bowl-size portion. Another day it may be just a salad of beets and chopped onion. This is still a seriously useful nutritional move.

Eat vegetables at both lunch and supper, and even as part of a snack if you can.

Fruit
Gettin' Down with Legal Sweets and Special Fibers

Imagine being out wandering the countryside, coming across a clump of wild strawberries on a warm sunny day. Maybe as you pass a stream, you find a bush full of blueberries, perfect for snacking. You sit down and munch away. Fruit and berries must be a regular part of your snacking routine. Your body has processed this sugar for tens of thousands of years. In cave people times, there were no bagels, crackers, cookies and cupcakes to snack on. Even modern inventions like whole wheat pretzels are second rate snacks in comparison.

So many fruits, and lots of time!

Fruit concepts

Here is a list of 25 fruits, to remind you of the many choices you have. Fresh, canned and dried all work.

- Frozen berries, blended with Whey protein powder, make excellent breakfast smoothies.
- Behind the scenes, fruit fibers keep intestinal cells in good shape. Eating fruit nurtures beneficial bacterial systems in the gut and all over the body.
- Try to eat fruit at least 3 times a day, maybe more. The fruits with an asterisk * have more pectin, which lowers cholesterol.
- Juices are missing the fiber and minerals of whole fruits. Many are made with apple or white grape juice concentrates: this means sugar-syrup. Have 4oz. servings of at most.
- Drink water or seltzer for thirst, and eat solid fruits for health.

Sources

Fruits in **bold type** have extra anti-oxidant value.

Apples*	Nectarines	*Dried Fruits: extra sweet*
Applesauce*	**Oranges**	Dates
Apricots	**Papaya**	Figs
Bananas*	Peaches	Raisins
Blackberries	Pears*	Cran-raisins
Blueberries	Pineapple	
Cantaloupe	Plums	*4 oz juices*
Clementines	**Pomegranate**	Apricot nectar
Grapefruit	**Raspberries**	Pineapple juice
Honeydew	**Red grapes**	Grapefruit juice
Kiwis	**Strawberries**	Orange juice
Lychee	Watermelon	
Mangos		

Consider this: you are the boss and are looking for cheap fuel for the workers building a pyramid in Egypt, or a great wall in China. Bread and rice do the trick. Grains have become popular in the past ten thousand years, but food for poor laborers is not what makes you the healthiest, though. The point of the story is that fruit is the ideal fuel for snacks; it is rich in minerals and vitamins. You will still have grains in your diet, but this is just an argument for why you need to be snacking on fruits, multiple times a day, then adding grains after that.

Another concept: all the pigments in fruit (and vegetables) have anti-oxidant properties. Eating more antioxidants translates into less stray electron damage in brain, liver, muscles and other places. The book *What Color Is Your Diet?* by David Heber, MD, Ph D. explains this idea more fully.[11] He's brilliant, and wants you to think red, orange, yellow, green, blue, etc.

Many people worry about bananas: whether their sweetness raises blood sugars too much. For people concerned about blood sugar responses, eat solid fruits, don't drink juices. Also, don't eat fruits and starches/grains at the same sitting. Having 100 calorie servings, even of dried fruits, generally won't excessively burden your blood sugar management system. Eat fruits with nuts, seeds, or protein, to slow their digestion, reducing the risk of quick surges in blood sugar. Berries, combined with nuts or seeds, were a routine part of daily fuel for hunters and gatherers.

Just a side note: when muscles are all warmed up from physical exercise, they absorb blood sugars more easily, and need less insulin to help process the sugar in the blood. Fruit snacks during walks and bike rides are perfect.

People in the olden days ate at least 4 or 5 servings of fruit a day, and stayed healthy. You do the same, to stay in a good state of repair.

Starches and Fat
Selecting Foods for Energy

You have read about protein for self-repair. You have read about fruits and vegetables to support enzymes and hormones that keep your body healthy. Now think about food for energy. The calories fueling your brain, your kidneys, your eyes, and your muscles comes from a mixture of starches and fats. Starches are foods like kidney beans, (sweet) potatoes, bread, noodles, pasta, crackers and rice. Starch plus grease and sugar equals muffins, cakes and cookies.

Fats come in avocado, nuts and seeds, and in oils. Fats are also found in spreads, like butter, margarine, and cream cheese. Fried foods, like French fries, potato chips and corn chips contain fats. You probably realize that there are some fat grams in the fish, chicken, meats and cheese you eat, too.

When it comes to how much to eat of fuel foods, think about your activity level. The average person, not getting much exercise or physical activity, needs to take it easy in the amount of fat and starch in his or her diet. If you are reading this

Starches

Providing carbohydrate fuel for brain and muscles

Here is a list of starches (carbohydrates). The foods in **bold type** in the chart on the next page are the best starches to be eating. They are dense with minerals. Eat less of the foods in the column labelled **Careful**: much of their nutrition has been processed out.

- Legumes and (sweet) potatoes give you a 3 to 4 times bigger amount of minerals like magnesium and potassium than do rice and pasta or even whole wheat bread.

- Starches, technically "hydrated carbons" get digested and become blood sugar. Starches that digest slowly are the best ones for keeping a slow, steady supply of energy coming into your brain and muscles.

- Notice that beans are a starch. Yes, they have some extra protein compared to grains, but only 7 grams protein per 1/2 cup. They are the ideal starch. Try to eat half a cup every day for their magnesium.

- "Eat more whole grains" (in the middle column) is a popular message. While these are better than white, processed grains, legumes and roots are still far more nutritious.

- More people get intestinal discomfort from eating wheat than anyone realizes, even whole wheat. The high gluten content in wheat irritates intestinal cells in many people. See reflux remedies pg. 105 for more details of this.

- Explore grains like rye, millet, quinoa and buckwheat: no excess hybridization.

—Continued on next page

Sources
Starches in **bold type** have extra anti-oxidant value.

Black beans	Barley	*Careful*
Black-eyed peas	Buckwheat	Bagels
Chickpeas	Cheerios	Cakes
Hummus	Corn	Candy
Lentils	Corn tortillas	Cookies
Lima beans	Millet	Muffins
Navy beans	Oat Bran	Noodles
Pinto beans	Oatmeal	Pancakes
Red kidney beans	Peas	Saltines
Sweet potatoes	Plantain	Spaghetti
White kidney beans	Potatoes	Waffles
Yams	Quinoa	White bread
	Rice	Whole wheat bread
100% Rye bread		

book, hopefully you are someone who gets a decent amount of physical activity. Starches and fat fuel muscles involved in both cardio and weight-lifting activity.

Whether carbohydrates are digested quickly or slowly is an important issue when eating for health. Quickly metabolized carbs trigger a bigger insulin response. The size of the insulin response translates to more or less of a "build fat" message in the body. Most people are trying to avoid that. Read more about this in the chapters on managing weight, triglycerides and diabetes.

Be Careful in Picking Your Starches

Sunlight beams down energy, linking carbon and water together, forming carbohydrates: hydrated carbon. We eat grains, roots, beans and fruits. After digestion, those hydrated bits of carbon travel to cells to be used for fuel. We extract the sunlight energy from the food, exhaling carbon dioxide and water vapor. It is a very elegant process.

Carbohydrates are important for helping maintain a good metabolic rate. Starch calories are also important for people who have a good fitness routine. After exercise, muscles need to replenish their glycogen (stored starch) levels, otherwise they won't have fuel to perform tomorrow. Low fuel levels leave people with a feeling of fatigue.

A bit of advice, don't get too swept away in the very low carbohydrate diet trend. Being careful of starches and carbs for a few months, as part of a weight loss effort is fine. The emphasis on significantly limiting carbs applies mostly to sedentary people with extra upper-body area fat (apple-shaped people) who are trying to lose weight. People carrying their extra weight below the belt, pear-shaped, should continue to enjoy carbs, and just walk off their stored fat. Eating a diet too low in carbohydrates for too long can slow down metabolism, meaning the body adapts to living with lower fuel intake.

Don't get too swept away in the very low carbohydrate diet trend.

True, some people still need to be careful of their carbohydrate servings at each meal or snack. Some people do have a thrift gene, which means they gain weight easily, and the weight accumulates in the mid-abdomen area. For these people, yes, watching carbohydrates does matter. Half the black women in America have that thrift gene[12] that converts carbs to fat for storage quickly. The same is true for many Hispanic people. Also, if you were once obese, and now trim, you have fat cells ready to ambush your carbohydrate calories to try to refill themselves. You'll want to keep your starch servings to a size that carefully matches your metabolic needs at the moment. See the diabetes and weight control sections for more help with this.

By the way, one other concept about the process of how sunlight energy is unlocked from our food to give us energy... a bit of the energy transfer does go haywire, and this is one source of the stray electrons called free radicals. Cleaning up stray electrons is an important activity in the body; otherwise the charged particles cause damage. Think of it as mini-sunburns in cells.

You Need to Know the *Fats* of Life!

You want to think about which fats are the natural ones that your body is most comfortable metabolizing. The fats found in fish are important to health; those in turkey and chicken are okay. For thousands of years, the fats in nuts and seeds have been the oils your body expected to encounter every day. Again, think back to the good old days, 30,000 years ago, when nuts and berries were the routine morning and afternoon snack. When eating nuts and seeds, a handful is one serving. Remember, you'd have to climb another tree to get a second handful.

You'd usually go looking for snacks easier to gather, so your diet was not overly fatty then. The elk, moose and bison you ate were lean too. Modern fats, like corn oil, vegetable oil, Crisco, beef fat and cheese fat, are harder for your body to deal with. An easy way to picture it: Crisco, beef and cheese fat are thick and make you dense too. Air does not get into your lungs as well. Blood doesn't get to your muscles as well. Brain cells become sluggish too.

The modern oils, like corn and vegetable, are too thin; they can make your system over-react to irritations. An example, if you have arthritis, the modern oils can make you feel more "itis." If you have hepatitis, your liver cells can be more irritated from eating too much modern fat. Basically, the unhealthy fats and oils enhance the baseline inflammation level in your body. Eating these fats counteracts what you are trying to do when you take ibuprofen or aspirin to squelch inflammation.[13]

If you are a person who already turns starch to fat in a hurry, eating more beef and cheese fat can make you even more likely to store fat. The presence of these fats in your system causes the release of greater amounts of insulin.[14] The fat from grass-fed cows and sheep, on the other hand, is fine. There is an omega-3 component to the fat. Even ice cream in the authentic Crete diet has omega-3 fats. This fact would make steak and cheese from grass-fed cows and sheep quite acceptable in a healthy diet.

The oils in fish, like salmon, sardines and herring, tell your body to try to burn off fat. They also turn down the "convert starch to fat" message. They are anti-inflammatory as well.[15] You probably know the term for these good fats: omega-3's. You likely know their code letters EPA (eicosapentaenoic acid) and DHA (docosapentaenoic acid).

The Good Fats Story Continues ...

In nature, there are omega-3 fats in plants, like seaweed, purslane, and other leafy greens. There are omega-3 fats in pecans and walnuts and ground flax seeds. There are some in canola and soy oils too. All the plant forms of omega-3 fats are termed alpha linolenic acid (ALA.) Only about 5% to 10% of the ALA omega-3's that humans eat will be transformed to the longer molecules we commonly call omega-3 fish oils eicosapentaenoic acid and docosahexaenoic acid abbreviated as EPA and DHA.[16]

I point out the difference, simply because all omega-3's don't act alike. They are all structurally useful, but it is the EPA and DHA forms that are much more potent when it comes to being anti-inflammation and anti-aging agents in the body. For instance, I don't want you thinking that the ground flax seeds dusted

Caveperson fats

Foraging for nuts and seeds

Fats that are still here from caveman times keep your body in good shape.

- For a while, the government nutrition message said all fat is bad. This was the wrong advice.
- Nut oils and fish oils keep your body slick and flexible. This is good for keeping your blood flowing well and your brain thinking sharply.
- Important: modern poly-unsaturated oils can cause excess inflammation. Avoid corn and vegetable oil.
- Dining tip: toss a tablespoon of nuts or seeds on your vegetables at supper, like walnuts on your spinach or pine nuts on cauliflower.
- Nuts (paired with fruit) are a smart snack in the afternoon for major health benefits.
- Butter from grass-fed cows is okay in modest amounts.

Sources

Nuts and seeds in **bold type** are extra fierce.

Almonds	**Chia seeds**	*Be modest*
Brazil nuts	**Ground Flax**	Butter (from grass-fed
Cashews	**seeds**	cows is best)
Hazelnuts	Hemp seeds	Lard
Macadamia nuts	Pepitas	
Peanuts	Pumpkin seeds	*Avoid*
Pecans	Sesame seeds	Canola oil
Pine nuts	Sunflower seeds	Corn oil
Pistachio nuts		Cottonseed oil
Soy nuts	Avocado	Cream cheese
Walnuts	Coconut oil	Fried fast foods
	Olives	Safflower oil
	Olive oil	Stick margarine
	Peanut oil	Vegetable oil

into your yogurt or salad will keep your lungs calm as a person with asthma, the way EPA/DHA in salmon, trout and fish oil pills will.[17] The ALA will not sooth arthritic joints either, fish and krill oils do help joints.

The fat that predominates in corn oil, vegetable oil, safflower oil, and even soy bean oil and most seeds is the omega 6 fat linoleic acid, code letters LA. Like the ALA omega-3, Omega 6's are transformed to longer length molecules in our bodies, becoming something called arachidonic acid (AA.) AA feeds the inflammation-generating agents called prostaglandins, like PGE_2 (pronounced prostaglandin E two).[18] People take aspirin and Motrin to stop PGE_2–induced inflammation activity.

A diet too high in omega 6 fats can result in excess PGE_2 inflammatory signals going through the body. Instead of risking side effects from non-steroidal agents like Motrin, Ibuprofen and Celebrex which are all pills taken to reduce PGE_2 production, deprive your system of inflammation-producing oils in your food.

Just a neat nutrition note, Andrew Stoll, MD, at Harvard University, is conducting studies where he is treating depression with 5 to 10 grams a day of supplemental omega-3 EPA/DHA fish oil (in pill form),[19] and people's moods are lifting. (See www.omegabrite.com for info.)

Speaking of omega-3 fish oils, in the Framingham Heart Study, people eating fish three times a week, had higher DHA levels in their blood, and cut their risk of senile dementia in half, compared to people with lower DHA levels.[20] Fish plus other elements in the Mediterranean diet seem to reduce rates of dementia.[21] When I encounter people who are lacto-ovo vegetarian and simply don't eat any fish, I tell them I am worried about their aging brain and its structural need for EPA/DHA. I encourage them to either consume some fish oil pills, or look into the DHA supplements that are made from an algae source.[22] There are "gummy fish" style candy supplements that contain algae-derived DHA.[23] Taking 180 mg a day of DHA would be a wise idea for people who do not eat fish routinely.

The risk of Alzheimer's disease goes up in people with lower levels of DHA in the brain, as does the risk of decline in eyesight.

A brilliant psychiatric researcher at NIH, Joseph Hibbeln MD, gives wonderful lectures on the topic of EPA/DHA deficiency and development of chronic disease. He has compared fish consumption in various countries with the assortment of health problems that arise in them. He points out that in Japan, the country with the highest consumption of EPA/DHA, heart disease, stroke, and depression rates are radically lower than in places like the USA or even Poland.[24] Dr. Hibbeln, in medical articles, also writes about the imbalance of omega 6 and omega-3 levels in our American diet, and the higher incidence of dyslexia, of hyperactivity disorders and even of the tendency to violence. He also cited a 2002 study showing that adding vitamins, minerals and omega-3 fatty acids to young adult British prisoners' diets reduced antisocial behavioral offenses by 37 percent in nine months.[25]

The nutritional science and metabolic concept to carry with you is that all cells in the body have a fat component to the membrane wall. How the cell operates, then, is a function of cell wall fat composition. A better omega-3 fat component of the cell wall has a beneficial impact on so many conditions. The list includes hypertension, heart disease, diabetes, arthritis, anxiety and depression.[26]

Your body evolved expecting you to be eating the oils found in fish, sometimes from birds, and maybe a little fat from a swift, lean animal. Toss in some nuts and seeds, and you get the full picture of the fats your ancestors experienced. Your brain cells especially want you eating essential EPA/DHA omega-3 fats.

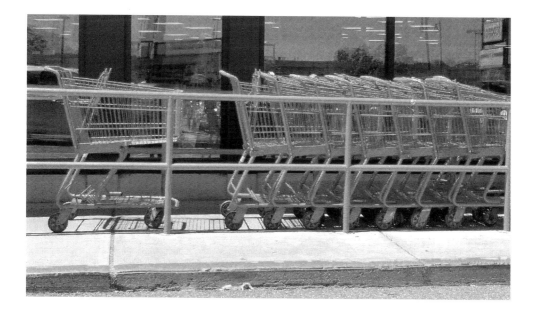

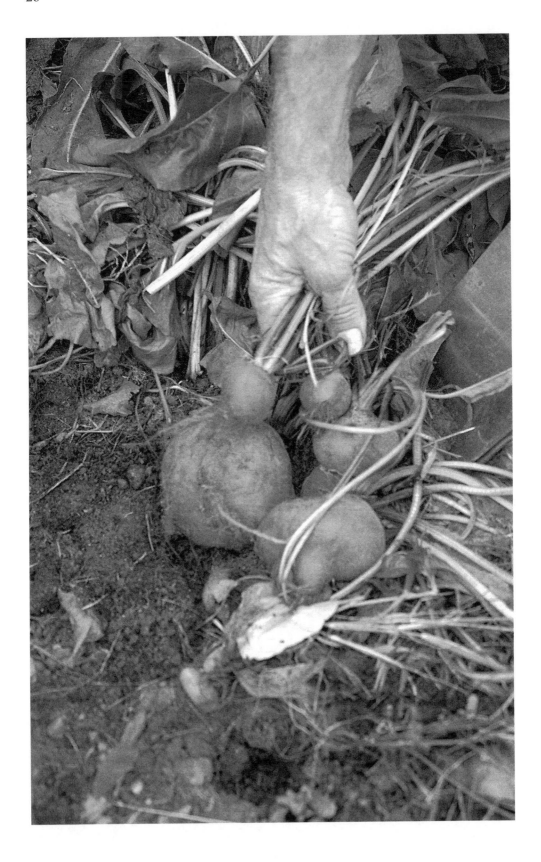

PART 2:

The Science and Physiology of Aging

… more nutrition, fewer meds.

What is really happening in your body as you age? Yes, your muscles recover more slowly; yes, it takes you longer to get over a cold. Are these events inevitable, or would your nutrient intake modify them? Read on.

More Drugs, but Healthier Aging? _____

I hope that some more science information will inspire or convince you to make even better food and lifestyle choices. Smoking, poor diet, and physical inactivity were the main causes of death for 35% of Americans over age 65 in year 2000 statistics. Clearly these three are behaviors that people can change.[27]

For a variety of reasons, people end up with conditions that require the use of prescription medicines. Use of these drugs is rising. While this may be for prevention of future trouble, or for managing current illness, there are consequences: the rising cost of health care, and the increasing incidence of adverse side effects to medicines. See *Table of Prescription Medication Use*[28] below.

Table of Prescription Medication Use

% Americans taking 1 Prescription/day

AGE GROUP	YRS. 1988-1994	2005 - 2008
45 – 64	54.8	64.8
65+	73.6	90.1

% Americans taking 3 or more prescriptions/day

AGE GROUP	YRS. 1988-1994	2005 - 2008
45 – 64	20.0	34.1
65+	35.3	65.0

All kinds of reasons account for the upsurge in drug-taking. A higher percentage of the population is getting health care. Treatment is more aggressive for hypertension, high cholesterol and osteoporosis. I see many people who are taking prescription drugs for their ailments, but don't particularly feel better. Rx pills may not be as dynamically effective as people and their medical providers think.

In looking at prescription drug effectiveness, there is a term, "number needed to treat" which means how many people will have to take a drug for there to be some usefulness for a single person. Example: in the "Statins to Lower Heart Attacks Trial" in Air Force people in Texas, 375 people with high cholesterol had to take the drug Lovastatin for 3 years before 1 person was protected from a heart attack or stroke.[29] Would you take a medicine if you had those odds of it being useful? Would you look for a more effective intervention to reduce your heart attack risk? A recurring theme here is that medicines are not as helpful as people think, and that lifestyle activities, while not as easy as taking pills, offer far more benefits.

I want people to investigate which of their ailments could be reversed with an expert blend of food, nutrition, fitness and energy healing modalities.

Insights into Food and Corrosion

Stray Electrons/Free Radicals

You have probably noticed, there is a wide range of how "old" someone looks or feels at a particular age. There are a few research doctors who look at what might be the reason for variable rates of aging. Dr. Stig Bengmark is a specialist in supporting the natural immune system. One of his particular interests is how to nourish the set of cells in the intestines that make antibodies to infections: gut-associated lymph tissue (GALT.) The friendly bacteria that live in our intestines, and the dietary fibers that nourish them, are the major support system for GALT. He looks at what might get in the way of having a healthy gut flora population. Prescription drugs, like Zantac and Nexium, disturb the gut flora, and of course antibiotics really cause trouble there. Smoking cigarettes and drinking excessive amounts of alcohol are problematic too. Eating more food fibers like the pectins in bananas, apples and pears nurtures the friendly gut microbes. See more on supporting gut flora in the acid reflux remedy section.

Beyond gut bugs, Dr. Bengmark is also looking at what food is doing to immune function and aging. He points out how the processing of food really disturbs key metabolism events in the body.[30] His particular concern is that excessive heating of foods causes inflammation in the body. Sugary components of food get somewhat caramelized and stick to proteins, and this causes irritations. The charming term for this reaction, is AGE: Advanced Glycation Endproducts. Examples of this kind of browning are the end parts of a roast beef when you roast it. In the body, it is the caramelized blood cell hemoglobin which is the Hemoglobin A1C test in diabetes. AGE then contributes to RAGE, which is activation of receptors for AGE. The chronic immune activation of RAGE causes immune dysfunction and speeds up aging.[31]

Inflammation is a primary mechanism behind basic aging, plus it accelerates

Alzheimers, atherosclerosis, and many cancers. In a simple way, inflammations are cell surfaces that are not repairing adequately. The electrons that are supposed to be maintaining the structural integrity of cell walls are spinning out of orbit. The electrons are then irritating neighboring cell membranes. For instance, take sunburns. The sun's energy can be too much for skin. A sunburn is just too many electrons jumping around the surface of the skin cells. It is the same concept for arthritis: excessive stray electrons on the bone surface in a joint leave the surface rough, and you hurting.

Besides taking medicines to reduce the inflammation rate in the joint, you want nutrients that will repair the bone surfaces, and get them back to being healthy. First, give some attention to avoiding food items that are unstable and irritating, or toxic to you or your bone surfaces. Then, some specialty nutrition may be needed, like more collagen. Your body can only repair a certain amount of "itis" in any given day. If it has to cope with unruly electrons in unstable modern fats like corn oil, plus the irritation of hybridized wheat, plus stray electrons of arthritic joints, something may get neglected. Usually it is your joints that suffer.

People in their 60's and 70's very often have a feeling that their medical conditions are just a fact of aging. They wind up taking an increasing number of prescriptions to manage these conditions they associate with aging. At some point, taking so many medicines can start to feel annoying and uncomfortable and sometimes futile.

Key Concept:

A major part of aging is really just irritated cells struggling to repair and losing their battle.

Remember, protein assembly does slow with aging, so it takes a little longer to repair brain cells, muscles and organs. Fierce nutrition is the best solution for slowing aging, and improving rehabilitation.

PART 3

Assembling a Food Plan

This chapter helps you map out the true details of what you can eat as meals and snacks to maximize your vitality.

What breakfast will help lower your blood pressure? What lunch soothes your joints? What supper can really fuel your brain?

The Right Amount Of Food

Understanding Fuel Needs

As you might imagine, genes, personality and lifestyle elements all contribute to your fuel needs. The response to stress is usually fat accumulation. The response to sleep deprivation is usually weight gain. Genes play a role in metabolism, but it's too late to pick new parents. You likely already have a sense of whether you have a slower or faster metabolism, as dictated by genetics. There is a section on weight control, that may help people who struggle with weight management, or who have athletic needs.

For now, think of fuel in two segments. There is energy you need to repair and restore your basic core self. This is the energy for your heart, your brain, your kidneys, your intestines, your liver and basic systems: your basal metabolism. Then you want to think about fuel for the physical activity aspect of your life. Obviously, different people have differing activity levels. Ballroom dance and yoga classes don't require as much fuel as what you would need for your daily, hour-long, jogging, swimming and cycling sessions.

Various body parts have different fuel needs. The brain runs on sugar. The heart runs on fats. The diaphragm runs on a mixture: half fat and half sugar. Arm and leg muscles run on a mixture that is about 80% starch and 20% fat, in general. Active people might like to know that after about 25 minutes of continuous aerobic effort, the arm and leg fuel mix can change, burning more like 50% to 60% fat.

> *To calculate your total fuel needs, think of your core body needs, then add on extra fuel for medical conditions, workouts or added recreational activities.*

An average metabolism for a person over 50 can be about 13 to15 calories per pound of ideal weight. We all know a few people who seem to eat tons of food, and stay amazingly thin. They are not the average person. The 13 to 15 calories number presumes that you are doing some modest physical movement each day, like housecleaning, walking 10 minutes to the bus stop and back each day, and maybe some occasional yard work. Add on the fuel needs of either coping with rheumatoid arthritis, or coping with labored breathing from COPD, and you figure another 1 to 2 calories per pound of what you weigh. You could guesstimate that 15- 17 calories per pound of ideal weight is a good figure for physiologically stressful situations.

After age 50, your metabolic systems may be slowing down. If you have a thyroid problem, your metabolism may be slower. If you've had multiple injuries, and are slowed up, you have to eat a little less. Some medicines also make the body convert food to fat more readily. Some people think of Type 2 diabetes as evidence of a thrift gene, sending any extra calories to fat cells for storage more readily. You may have to adjust the calorie level down one or two percentage points because of these conditions.

More Calories For Physical Activity

Keeping yourself in good physical health is one of the more pro-active steps you could take as you age. Think about it: your heart pumps more strongly, and the extra blood flow delivers more oxygen and nutrients to the nooks and crannies of your body. More antioxidants come with the flow as well. Doing 30 minutes of physical activity almost daily is a key component of mental and physical wellbeing. It is a good move to help feel more confident that you'll maintain good health in your later years.

If you are living an active lifestyle, give yourself some extra fuel when you do more workouts. On a Sunday, a two-hour bike ride might burn up 600 to 800 to 1000 calories, depending on your pace and intensity. Let's say you think of your core 160 lb. self, needing 2400 calories (160 x 15) and then you add on 600 calories for your 2 hour ride; you may need to eat 3000 calories so that you'll feel restored the next day. This is not a "must eat" message, but I mention it for people who may be trying to do more exercise on a consistent basis, and I want them to repair and re-energize adequately each day. See the weight control section for how to cut back on calories when still doing a good amount of physical activity.

Use the diagram on the next page to understand what your muscles are using for fuel when you are exercising.

When pedalling a bike or walking briskly, you start out burning about 80% glycogen (starch) and 20% triglyceride (fat) as the fuel mix in your muscles. Once warmed up, the mix is about 50-50. The fuel shift occurs about 25 minutes into the activity. Here is a weight control tip: if you want to eat some extra pizza and pasta calories and not gain weight, exercise a bit longer before the meal, then there will be room for the carbohydrate calories in your muscles, otherwise the carbs get converted to fat and sent to fat cells. Also notice in the diagram that in sprinting, muscles go back to starch-burning. If you are trying to lose weight,

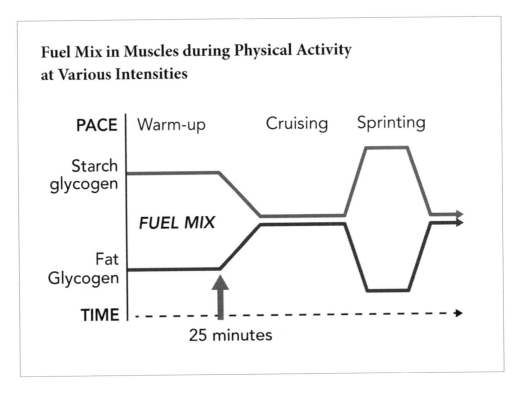

Fuel Mix in Muscles during Physical Activity at Various Intensities

don't push so hard that you are gasping for air. This means you are not getting enough oxygen to burn fat.

When thinking about eating starches, a big focus is on how the hormone insulin responds to your meals. Insulin is a "move sugar" message in the body, telling cells to open up and let sugar, a product of digested starches, fruits and juices, into muscles where the carbohydrate calories are needed for fuel. Insulin also has "build fat", "retain sodium", and "make hungry" messages. If you are working on weight loss, or managing blood fats (triglycerides), clearly you want to keep insulin messaging lower. To accomplish this, you would eat smaller portions of starches, and select the ones that digest slowly.

Also, it happens that warm muscles need less insulin to process sugars. If you're worried about weight, and have the urge to eat some extra cereal, potatoes or pasta, eat these extra carbs just after your brisk walk or bike ride. After exercise, there is room in the muscles for the carb calories you want, plus there won't be as much of a "build fat" insulin message sending the carbs to fat cells instead.

One other important component of your daily fuel needs is your muscle mass – the total amount of muscle you have on your bones. As people age, they may do less physical activity so their muscles shrink in volume, as well as in strength. Again, the term for this muscle loss is sarcopenia.

Weight-lifting Activity is Important
Maintaining Muscle Volume

Maintaining your body's muscle volume plays out in many physical and mental areas in the body. It lowers your diabetes risk, it prevents heart attacks, and of course it means you get to enjoy a few more calories as well.

In his book *Biomarkers*,[32] Bill Evans looks at how maintaining muscle fitness and volume actually lowers your "biological age". It is a great read about the ways that physical fitness keeps you feeling and acting younger even while your years advance.

Eating adequate amounts of protein every day also matters to muscle integrity. Subtle deficiencies in protein over some years can lead to a substantial loss in muscle cell volume: sarcopenia. The muscles may only appear to have shrunk just a little bit in size, but what has also taken place is that fat deposits have replaced proteins inside muscle tissue, so there is much less strength. There will also be a change in how much food (calories) you get to eat, without gaining weight. Fat is low maintenance stuff, while protein-rich muscle fibers need more calories and nutrients to stay functional.

Establishing and maintaining some routine fitness activity isn't easy for some people. Do whatever it takes to keep your head in the game, though. Maybe it is an "exercise class for people with arthritis" at a local senior center. For maintaining your muscle volume and strength, find a local gym or other facility, like the "Y", that has classes or equipment. Daytime hours at local gyms have more and more retirees in attendance. There's no need to be lifting barbells; you can be using simple machines.

For truly productive fitness activity, the parameters to consider are the amount of weight to lift, and how many repetitions. You might start with one well-known authority, The American College of Sports Medicine, http://acsm.org/docs/current-comments/resistancetrainingandtheoa.pdf. They provide general advice and precautions. Of all places, the site www.bodybuilding.com has some excellent information for basic muscle toning too. Get some help learning what these exercises are. Try them twice a week, for 3 or 4 weeks. See how you look and feel! This is their chart that may help you record your fitness activity.

Bodybuilding.com's Workout Log

Senior Fitness Beginners Exercise Program

Instructions: Under the "Set #__", fill in the weight you used and the number of reps you performed. The numbers beside each exercise
represent the number of sets and repetitions.

EXERCISE	SUGGESTED	SET #1	SET #2
Lat pulldown:	2x15	_____	_____
Leg press:	2x15	_____	_____
Chest press:	2x15	_____	_____
Seated leg curl:	2x15	_____	_____
Seated shoulder press:	2x15	_____	_____
Leg extension:	2x15	_____	_____
Bicep curl:	2x15	_____	_____
Tricep extension:	2x15	_____	_____
Abdominal crunches:	2x20	_____	_____

You will need to support your muscle-toning activity with enough protein in your diet. If you're under-eating, you'll just feel more tired, rather than invigorated and fit from your muscle-toning efforts.

To decide your total fuel needs, think of your core body needs, then add on extra fuel for medical conditions, workouts or added recreational activities.

How Much Protein Will You Need Each Day?
Hint: More Than You Thought.

Recent research in people over 60 is showing that protein needs may be much higher than previously thought. The added protein is for maintaining muscle mass. You know about osteopenia, the thinning/shrinking of bones with age. Even more important is "sarcopenia", the scientific word for loss of muscle mass. Less muscle means less strength, which can translate to a greater likelihood of falling when a person becomes frail. Why and how muscle is lost with age is not clear. It may be the result of a reduced capacity for turning dietary protein into muscle.[33] It may be that people are not using their muscles strenuously enough as they age, and therefore muscle mass dwindles.[34]

By age 60, half the population is showing signs of significant muscle loss, and almost 10% have limited mobility as a result.[36]

After about age 50, *i.e.,* as the body ages, research suggests people need to eat about 3/4 of a gram of protein for each pound of ideal weight. The calculation: multiply your ideal weight in pounds times ¾ or .75 to get the amount of protein in grams needed daily. If eating higher amounts of protein feels difficult, then spread out the protein intake over all three meals. Remember, eating protein at breakfast is good for your metabolism, and is a nice way to be sure you'll squeeze in all that you need each day. A minimum of 20 grams protein at any meal is what's needed to stimulate protein synthesis and prevent sarcopenia.[35] Also, in meeting the ¾ gram protein-per-pound of ideal weight goal, a third to half of the allotment should be plant-based. This requires significant quantities of protein from black beans, hummus and other legumes, and from vegetables and nuts, in the mix of your daily cuisine.

An older 150 lb. person certainly needs 75 grams of protein a day, and on up to 112 grams of protein is even better. Some people think, "Too much protein is not good for bones or kidneys or liver;" however, this thinking is out of date. Another outmoded idea to dispel is that eating two eggs for breakfast every day is unhealthy. In a group of weight-lifting 61-year-old people, raising dietary cholesterol intake from an average of 213 mg each day to 610 mg per day, by adding eggs, dairy foods and lean protein did not raise cholesterol numbers at all.[36]

Protein Content of Common Foods

AMOUNT	FOOD ITEM	PROTEIN (GRAMS)
8 oz	Milk (whole, skim, 1%, 2%)	8
8 oz	Soymilk	5+
1/2 cup	Low-fat Cottage Cheese	14
1 oz	Sliced Cheese	6+
1 Tbsp	Parmesan Cheese, grated	2
8 oz	Yogurt (regular, low fat, non fat)	8+
4 oz	Frozen Yogurt	2+
1 scoop	Whey Protein Powder	~17
1	Egg, Whole	6
1	Egg, White Only	3.5
4 oz	Salmon/Tuna, canned	26
4 oz	Fish, Chicken, Turkey, Pork, Beef	28
1/2 cup	Tofu	10
4 oz	Tempeh (aged tofu)	17
1	Soyburger	10+
1/2 cup	Chickpeas, Lentils, Black or Kidney Beans	7
1/4 cup	Hummus	6.5
2 Tbsp	Peanut Butter	8
4 Tbsp	Walnuts, Almonds, Cashews, Sunflower seeds	7
1 cup	Broccoli or Spinach, cooked	5
1/2 cup	Peas	4
1 cup	Pasta	7
1/2 cup	Quinoa, cooked volume	5
1	Baked Potato, large	4
1 cup	Rice	4
1 cup	Ready-to-eat Cereal: Cheerios, Nutrigrain	4
1	English Muffin	4
2 slices	Bread, whole grain	4
1	Sports Bar (Balance Bar, Power Bar)	10+

Use this table for ideas on reaching 20-30 grams protein at each meal. Notice how nuts, seeds and beans can be helpful. Again, there is no need to neglect eggs.

As you're thinking about protein foods, I want to emphasize how useful eating one serving of oily fish per week is. This could reduce risk of sudden cardiac death by 50%, and help people live longer in general.[37] Yes, a fish oil pill works too, if you simply don't eat fish.

People in caveperson times got about a third of their calories from protein.[38] Remember this was all the correct proteins; there were no other options. Even the flesh of grass-fed deer and antelope is nice lean protein, and rich in the Omega-3 fats that we now think of just in fish.

It is so important that people start to consume fish rich in Omega-3 fats more frequently. Here is a simple recipe. Costco and Trader Joe's sell canned, wild Alaskan salmon. Skinless pink salmon, sprinkled with lemon juice, is as mild as tuna. It's low cost, and no worries about mercury and PCPs in these relatively smaller, wild fish.

Instead of your usual tuna sandwich, make a wild salmon salad. Try the recipe on the next page to see if this is works for you.

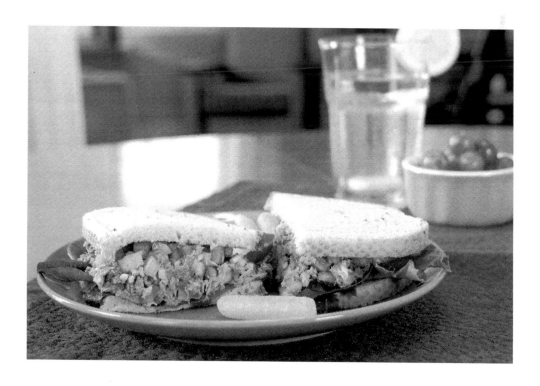

Salmon Salad

Ingredients

1 6-ounce can wild Alaskan salmon

2-3 stalks chopped celery

1-2 Tbsp balsamic vinegar

(Paul Newman's balsamic vinaigrette salad dressing works well too.)

Optional additions:

2-3 Tbsp dill pickles, chopped

2-3 Tbsp chopped mild onion

½ cup cannellini (white) beans

Directions

Mix all ingredients and serve on salad greens, or on rye bread or rye crackers.

Serves 1 or 2 people, depending on size and hunger.

What Would an Incredibly Nourishing Diet Look Like?

As I have said before, a serious intake of vegetable, fruits and legumes is the cornerstone of the Mediterranean (Crete) diet.

The government puts out recommendations for minimal quantities of fruits and vegetables to consume for basic nourishment. These government numbers don't reflect caveman era intake, but they are a good start for supporting health. I list the number here so you can decide if you are doing pretty well, or could improve.

Let me translate the numbers into simple behaviors you can focus on.

1) Eat a serving of fruit three times a day, meaning 21 servings a week.
2) Eat at least 2 cups of vegetables (cooked volume) a day. One box of frozen vegetables is about 2 cups, or 11 ounces by weight.

These are the key minimum amounts to eat. How does your routine cuisine stack up? These are not easy target number to meet. It takes a commitment to shopping more frequently and really planning meals and snacks until they become good habits.

The standard easy offerings at fast food places and lunch counters don't support vibrant vegetable and fruit ingestion. You often have to carry a certain amount of snacks with you each day to reach the target numbers.

Dietary Guidelines for Americans, 2016

Fruit and Vegetable Recommendations

People, age 51+ years

FOODS	WOMEN	MEN
Fruits, cups per day	1.5	2.0
Vegetables, cups per day	2.0	2.5
Vegetable assortment, cups per week		
Dark Green	1.5	2.0
Red & Orange	4.0	5.5
Beans & Peas	1.0	1.5
Starchy Vegetables	4.0	5.0
Legumes	1.5	1.5

Sample Food Plans

These next few pages offer sample daily menus to summarize what eating the right amount of protein, fruit, vegetables and legumes would look and feel like. Daily intake is 13 – 15 calories per pound of ideal weight. So a trim, 120-pound person may look at the 1800 calories menu.

Everyone has varying tastes, so these can be modified, and there is always a dessert cookie to add sometimes too. These are just the core plans.

A food plan for someone who should weigh 125–130 lbs.
~1800 calories

MEAL	FOOD	CALORIES
BREAKFAST		
protein:	2 oz turkey, 3 Tbsp protein powder or 1/2 cup cottage cheese	100
fruit:	a small banana, 3/4 cup fresh or canned fruit	80
nuts:	1 Tbsp peanut butter or handful of nuts or seeds	100
dairy:	6 oz no-fat yogurt or 8 oz skim milk	80
beverage:	(optional) coffee, regular or green tea	
SNACK		
starch	1 granola bar, 1.5 cup Cheerios or 1 cup oatmeal	150
or fruit:	a small box of raisins or 10 dried apricot halves	
beverage:	4 oz skim milk, or a few Tbsp yogurt	40
LUNCH		
protein:	3 oz salmon, sardines, turkey, chicken or lite cheese	150
starch:	1/2 cup kidney beans or lentils or 1 cup peas or corn	150
veges:	2 lg carrots, or a tomato and a green pepper	60
SNACK		
Dairy:	8 oz skim milk or 6 oz light yogurt	80
SNACK		
nuts:	1 handful (2 Tbsp) walnuts, cashews, or sunflower seeds	100
fruit:	a lg peach, 3/4 cup pineapple chunks, or 1 med. apple	75
DINNER		
protein:	4 oz broiled fish, seafood, poultry, or lean meat	200
starch:	1 cup green peas, corn, limas, yam or baked potato	150
veges:	2 cups broccoli, cauliflower, spinach, carrots, etc.	80
oil:	1 Tbsp nuts, 2 tsp butter or 1 tsp olive oil	45
SNACK		
fruit:	a big orange or apple, 2 cup berries, or 2 plums or kiwis	100
dairy:	8 oz lite cocoa, 2 oz lite cheese or 1 cup low-fat yogurt	100

	Total calories:	**1840**

Extra munch:	1 quart lite popcorn, 2 cookies or a scoop of lite ice cream	100

Remember to take a better-than-average multivitamin with this food plan.

A food plan for someone who should weigh 150–165 lbs.
~2300 calories

MEAL	FOOD	CALORIES
BREAKFAST		
protein:	3 oz turkey,1/3 cup whey protein or 3/4 cup cottage cheese	130
fruit:	a large banana, or 1 cup peaches, pineapple or pears	120
nuts:	3 Tbsp walnuts, pecans, or sunflower seeds	135
dairy:	8 oz non-fat yogurt or 8 oz low fat milk	120
beverage:	(optional) coffee, regular or green tea	
SNACK		
starch or fruit:	1 cup (ckd vol) oatmeal, or 1.5 cup Cheerios or a granola bar a small box of raisins or 10 dried apricot halves	150
beverage:	(optional) green or regular tea or seltzer	
LUNCH		
protein:	4 oz salmon, sardines, turkey or lean ham	200
starch:	3/4 cup beans or lentils, 1.5 cup peas, or 2 slices rye bread	225
veges:	3 lg carrots, or 2 tomatoes and a green pepper	75
beverage:	seltzer w/ lime or iced tea	
SNACK		
nuts:	1 handful (3 Tbsp) walnuts, almonds, cashews, peanuts	150
fruit:	a lg. peach, 1 cup pineapple chunks, or a small mango	100
SNACK		
sweet:	2 Paul Newman's no-wheat fig newton cookies	100
DINNER		
protein:	6 oz broiled fish, poultry, tofu or lean pork	300
starch:	1 cup peas, corn, limas, baked potato, or small yam	150
veges:	2 cup broccoli, cauliflower, spinach, Swiss chard, etc.	80
oil/nuts:	2 Tbsp cashews, or ~1 Tbsp flax seeds , or 2 tsp olive oil or 2 tsp butter	90
SNACK		
fruit:	a medium orange or apple, 1 cup berries, or 1 pear	75
dairy:	8 oz skim milk or 6 oz no-fat yogurt	100

	Total calories:	**2300**

Remember to take a better-than-average multivitamin with this food plan.

A food plan for someone who should weigh 190–200 lbs.
~2800 calories

MEAL	FOOD	CALORIES
BREAKFAST		
protein:	3 oz turkey, 4 Tbsp whey protein or 1 cup cottage cheese	150
fruit:	a large banana, a grapefruit, or 2 clementines	120
nuts:	1/4 cup walnuts, pecans, Brazil nuts or sunflower seeds	175
dairy:	1 cup no-fat yogurt or 8 oz low fat milk	120
beverage:	black coffee, regular tea or green tea (optional)	
SNACK		
starch	1 cup oatmeal, 1.5 cup Cheerios, or a granola bar	150
or fruit:	1 small box raisins, 5 whole dried apricots or 2 med. apples	
beverage:	green tea, regular tea or water (optional)	
LUNCH		
protein:	4 oz salmon, turkey, chicken, or lean ham	200
starch:	3/4 cup kidney beans or lentils or 2 slices 100% rye bread	200
veges:	3 carrots, or 2 tomatoes and a green pepper	75
dairy:	8 oz low fat milk or fruit juice	140
sweet:	2 wheat-free fig newton cookies or 2 sm almond macaroons	100
beverage:	water or seltzer or iced tea	
SNACK		
nuts:	1 handful (3 Tbsp) walnuts, cashews or peanuts	150
fruit:	a lg. peach, 1 cup pineapple chunks, or a big apple	100
DINNER		
protein:	8 oz broiled fish, poultry, or lean meat	400
starch:	1.5 cups green peas, corn, limas, baked potato	225
veges:	2 cups broccoli, cauliflower, spinach, carrots, etc.	80
oil/nuts:	1 Tbsp olive oil, 3 Tbsp salad dressing or 3 Tbsp nuts	135
SNACK:		
fruit:	a huge orange or apple, or 2 plums	100
dairy:	8 oz skim milk or 6 oz no-fat yogurt	100
starch:	1.5 cup Cheerios; 1 cup oatmeal, or 5 cup lite popcorn	150
	Total calories:	**2855**

Remember to take a better-than-average multivitamin with this food plan.

PART 4

Smart Supplements ...

The line of reasoning that supports nutritional supplements

There is a popular saying, "If you eat a good diet, you don't need to take any vitamins." It is a nice thought, but no one ever really tested its validity. In other words, "show me the data". A number of studies now prove a significant depletion of nutrients from agricultural soils over the past 50 years, with a subsequent drop in nutrient content of both fruit and vegetables, plus chicken and beef. For example, an analysis from a composite group of 27 vegetables has shown a 24% drop in magnesium content during the period 1940 to 1991.[39][40]

In modern America, are we seeing examples of nutritional deficiency diseases? Are there are elements of the Paleolithic diet, missing from our modern diets, now causing negative health consequence? Could taking some dietary supplements compensate for those missing nutrients?

Consider this example: National surveys suggest that vitamin C deficiency can be found in at least 10% of the population, particularly the elderly. One case reported a man evaluated in an emergency room for pain that did not respond to narcotics. Further examination revealed the he suffered from scurvy, a disease caused by a deficiency of vitamin C.[41]

What would "sub-clinical" nutrient deficiencies look like? We think of heart disease as a cholesterol problem, or depression and violence as simple mental health issues. Some Omega-3 fish oil researchers see them all as evidence of a deficiency of dietary EPA/DHA Omega-3 fatty acids though.[42] In countries with much more Omega-3's in their diet, there is not as much depression or heart disease.

Something about the B vitamins

A number of conditions do seem to point to subtle nutritional deficits as a part of their development. Carotid artery stenosis, (the narrowing of the arteries in the neck that lead up to the brain), can result from modest B-vitamin deficiencies over time, according to research at the world famous Framingham Heart Study.[43] In a study watching 500,000 Europeans, higher blood levels of B vitamins and folic acid seemed to reduce the risk of lung cancer by 50%, even showing benefits in smokers.[44] Just so you know, we get less B vitamins in our diet than our ancestors did, because we are not eating moldy bugs, grubs and mushrooms from stumps any more. Many of my patients report having more daily energy once they start the multivitamins I recommend which include a good dose of B vitamins.

The Case For Magnesium

National surveys detect that most Americans are eating only about 2/3 of the recommended dietary intake --RDI -- for magnesium. Current intake is 50% lower than the amount we ate in the early 1900's.[45] What could the consequences be? While not many people show up with low blood levels of magnesium, subtle deficiencies inside cells are associated with more cholesterol sticking to artery walls, i.e., more rapid progression of atherosclerosis, leading to heart disease. The "subclinical deficiency of magnesium leads to impaired bone calcification, speeding up the development of osteoporosis. Low-level magnesium leads to more accumulation of fat in the stomach area.[46] Just an FYI note: drinking alcohol causes more loss of magnesium in urine, a mechanism behind the development of beer gut.[47] If you're not eating a half-cup of kidney or other beans, or 4 ounces of salmon today, or having 1/3 cup of seeds daily, you are likely not ingesting as much magnesium as you need. Seeds and legumes are

Highest Magnesium content foods

Magnesium RDI for people over age 50:
Females 320mg; Males 420mg

AMOUNT	FOOD ITEM	MAGNESIUM (MG)
1/4 cup	Pumpkin seeds	185
1/4 cup	Sunflower seeds	127
1/4 cup	Almonds	98
1/4 cup	Cashew pieces	88
2 Tbsp	Flax seeds	70
1 cup cooked	Soy beans	147
1 cup cooked	Black beans	120
1 cup cooked	Lima beans	81
1 cup cooked	Lentils	71
1 cup cooked	Green peas	62)
1 cup cooked	Brown rice	84
2 slices	Whole wheat bread	48
1 medium	Banana	32
1 medium	Orange	19

not a routine component of most people's diet preferences or habits now, so I'd like to see people take a multi-vitamin-multi-mineral pill that includes 100mg magnesium.

The More Vitamin D You Have, the Sunnier You Feel

Another nutrient for which diet may not provide sufficient amounts is vitamin D. Many centuries ago, sunlight shining on exposed skin generated most of our vitamin D; dietary vitamin D was just bonus material. Vitamin D in the blood ranges from about 30 to 100 nanograms/milliliter (ng/ml), or 50 to 140 nanomoles/liter (mmol/L) This "normal" range is set to account for 90% of the population. However, deficiency symptoms show up at levels below 32 ng/ml, and under 20ng/ml is very serious.

Eminent researcher Dr. Michael Hollick suggests optimal vitamin D range of 50 to 70 ng/ml or 115 to 128 nmol/l.[48] People in the upper 25% of the range are maintaining strong bones; people with blood levels of vitamin D in the lower 75% of the range are experiencing slow, subtle bone loss.[49] We most often think about vitamin D and bones but it matters to muscle volume as well. The number associated with healthier muscles is 60 nmol/l.[50] The classic vitamin D deficiency disease is rickets, and incidence of that is rare in the US. Osteomalacia is a softening of the bones due to low vitamin D intake. Let me also point out that the symptoms of osteomalacia are skeletal pain and muscle weakness. There are case reports where people complaining of painful bone aches went through the stress of cancer evaluation, because physicians don't think of vitamin D deficiency as capable of generating such bone pain.[51] All in all, have your blood levels of vitamin D checked as part of your routine health care. Again, above 30 ng/ml is a good number, but above 50 ng/ml is likely better.

More recent research data suggests that when vitamin D levels are lower, the immune system won't work at its best. Multiple sclerosis[52] and certain cancers occur more often in people with vitamin D in the lower parts of the normal range.[53] For most people, taking 1,000 units a day is the minimum suggested dose to reduce risk of deficiencies and disease.[54] I know of many people taking 4000 iu a day to maintain good levels through the Winter in the Boston area.

Vitamin D and The Flu

Vitamin D supplements for prevention of the flu have been a big research topic over the past decade or so. First, the true benefit of getting a flu shot is something of an unknown. A quote from the journal *Lancet Infectious Disease:*

> Recent excess mortality studies were unable to confirm a decline in influenza-related mortality since 1980, even as vaccination coverage increased from 15% to 65%.[55]

It is possible the vaccine helps small children and the frail and elderly. However, being older and frail are the main reasons that the vaccine doesn't generate antibodies to the viruses it hopes to prevent.

Meanwhile, vitamin D is emerging as a possibly strong agent for reducing the risk of contracting the flu. First, notice that the flu seems to happen in the darker months of the year in the northern latitudes, and in the rainy season in tropical regions.[56] There is also data that shows people get more respiratory infections and the flu as their vitamin D levels go down in Fall and Winter.[57]

Direct flu prevention trials using vitamin D in older adults have not yet happened. However, in several other studies where subjects were taking either 2000 iu of vitamin D per day or a placebo, both anecdote[58] and data[59] show significant reductions in illness occur. There is one study showing that 1200 iu/day vitamin D prevents flu in school children.[60] A note of caution: many studies claim no benefit from vitamin D in flu prevention, but the study designs were bad. There was no testing to see how deficient the study subjects were in vitamin D to begin with, and the trial supplement dose was generally too low to have any therapeutic effect.

> *… vaccine effectiveness, defined as the reduction in attack rates between vaccinated and unvaccinated population, expected to be between 70% and 90% in younger adults is considerably reduced to less than 40% over the age of 65 years…* [55]

Could better nutrition help a flu shot be fore effective? That idea has only been slightly studied. A trial using a supplement drink with a basic multivitamin and some extra antioxidants plus the immune-boosting mineral selenium along with a flu shot suggested there could be slight benefit.[61] Going as high as 200 iu vitamin E per day can improve the antibody response to other vaccines, particularly diptheria, tetanus and hepatitis B vaccines.[62] Taking a multivitamin that includes 200 iu vitamin E is something discussed later.

Vitamin D also seems to have a role in regulating cholesterol levels, where more vitamin D helps HDL (good) cholesterol numbers be higher, and LDL (bad) cholesterol numbers be lower.[63]

Cysteine
We're Just Not Eating Fur and Feathers Like We Used to!

One more example of diet being weak in a nutrient with subtle but significant consequences is the case of the amino acid cysteine. In the olden days we ate all sorts of critters, chewed 'em right up, fur, feathers and all. As a result, our diet naturally provided more of the sulfur-containing amino acid cysteine. Cysteine is the amino acid that is most crucial for the production of glutathione (GSH), the major antioxidant and detoxification enzyme in the body. GSH supports the repair of liver, lung and kidney cells. Glutathione also keeps eyes healthy, and prevents red blood cell damage from stray electrons, those free radicals I mentioned earlier. Glutathione also helps insulin function at its best. Maybe most importantly, the glutathione enzyme has a lot to do with immune system regulation and function. When glutathione enzyme levels run low, the immune system struggles.[64]

Cysteine supplements used to be the remedy for bronchitis, in the era before antibiotics and steroids, and they still have a role to play in modern times.[65] A large European clinical trial found that cysteine supplements, 600mg per day, were not of much benefit to people already taking steroids for their chronic obstructive lung disease (COPD). However, it was useful for people not medicated with steroids.[66] Well, people on continuous steroid therapy for lung issues should know that there is a significant increase in risk of cataracts as a side effect of that treatment.[67] Why not try nutrition therapy with cysteine first, to see how much you benefit. Avoid the risk of eye damage.

The reason for mentioning cysteine now, is that better glutathione levels mean less health glitches in older people.[68] All the proteins we eat have a little bit of cysteine in them but whey protein is the best food source. This is why I suggest whey as the protein people have in the morning. The beneficial bacteria that live in the intestines also produce key vitamins, and amino acids: particularly cysteine and L-glutamine.[69] So we're back to the importance of diet, and especially the fiber types, that will nurture the best array of beneficial microbes in the intestines.

This cysteine story illustrates an important point of this book. Make sure you are nourished first, then utilize medicines as needed. Prescription drug treatments for medical conditions may feel good in the short run because they are so fast acting, but may have negative effects in the long run. Andrew Weil, MD, points out in his book *Spontaneous Healing*, that people with arthritis who use ibuprofen and other non-steroidal anti-inflammatory agents for treatment, usually have a faster deterioration in joint health, than do people who make diet, exercise and lifestyle adjustments that nurture their joint surfaces.[70] We give antibiotics to treat an infection, so the drugs smack down the bug, but the body does the work of healing. How many subtle elements in the modern diet are missing and we therefore don't repair or heal as well?

Here is an example where modern life butts up against our altered food style, and repair systems struggle. Cave people didn't have fly ash (smog) and urban air pollution to contend with in their lungs, but if they did, they would have had plenty of cysteine to support the glutathione clean up system in their lungs. Today the situation is the opposite. We have more air pollution, but no one is consuming as much cysteine. Asthma rates are on the rise, so we know many people have lung cells that are struggling to repair, but they aren't eating the best repair nutrients.[71] There is a deficiency of antioxidants in people with asthma.[72] The number of Americans eating an adequate amount of antioxidant fruits and vegetables per day to be nourished is 10% to 30%, depending on how the adequacy is measured. One good fact though is that married seniors, men over 45 and women over 65 do better than most people, according to Neilson surveys.[73]

Don't Believe Any Bad News About Vitamin E

Another example of Paleo nutrition versus nutrient intake now is the case for vitamin E. Cave people ate the equivalent of 5 or 6 bags of leaves every day, like spinach, chard, beet greens, water cress, arugula, etc. Between the greens and the couple of handfuls of nuts and seeds they ate each day, they enjoyed much more vitamin E.[74] In the usual American diet now, people consume only 8 to 10 units of vitamin E per day. Is anyone suffering from vitamin E deficiency disease? The vision problems, anemia, and weakness that happen from true vitamin E deficiency are not evident here in America. There may be more subtle consequences of low intake though. In the Nurses Health Study conducted at Harvard University School of Public Health, women consuming 100 units a day of vitamin E (the average Paleolithic era intake) reduced their risk of heart disease by one third.[75] By the way, a similar one-third reduction in risk of heart failure occurs in people with Paleolithic levels of vitamin C intake, according to a very recent nutritional study.[76]

The point to appreciate is that super nourished people generally don't deteriorate at the same rate as most people currently do. Medicines are frequently just a balm on a wound that really would best benefit from nutritionally fueled healing. Despite the rigors of living in the wild, ancient people had good health.[77] Much thought-provoking information on this topic is found on The Weston Price Foundation website.[78]

Anthropologists report that the caveman era Paleolithic diet was rich in vitamins C and E, and the minerals zinc, magnesium and calcium, plus omega-3 fats. They consumed these nutrients in amounts much higher than anyone ever eats now. Eating more of these key nutrients is associated with absence of diseases.[79]

So You Really *Zinc* You're Eating Well, Huh?

Zinc is an important element when it comes to immune function. In a simple way, it gives immune cells sharper teeth for chewing up germs. It also matters a lot to skin repair and wound healing. Digestive enzymes are not released without zinc there to initiate the process. It also has a role in preventing acid reflux and reducing the risk of macular degeneration. The dietary reference intake (DRI) for Zinc is 8 mg for females, and 11 mg for males. Only 55% of the country eats a number that is even 75% of the DRI amount.[80] The best food sources of zinc are listed below. If you are not eating several foods from this list each day, your intake is likely below ideal. Once again, a vitamin-mineral supplement may be crucial to getting a healthy intake.

Best food sources for Zinc

AMOUNT	FOOD ITEM	ZINC (MG)
3 oz/wt	Oysters	20+ mg
3 oz/wt	Roast beef	9.0 mg
1 oz/wt	Alaskan King Crab	6.5 mg
1 cup	Baked beans	3.5 mg
1 oz/wt	Pumpkin seeds	3.0 mg
1 oz/wt	Squash seeds	3.0 mg
3 oz/wt	Chicken leg	2.7 mg
3 oz/wt	Pork tenderloin	2.5 mg
1 cup	Green peas	1.9 mg
1 oz/wt	Dry Roast Cashews	1.5 mg
½ cup	Chickpeas	1.3 mg
3 oz/wt	Chicken breast	1.0 mg
1 oz/wt	Dark 85% Chocolate	1.0 mg
1 oz/wt	Dry roast peanuts	1.0 mg
1 oz/wt	Almonds	1.0 mg

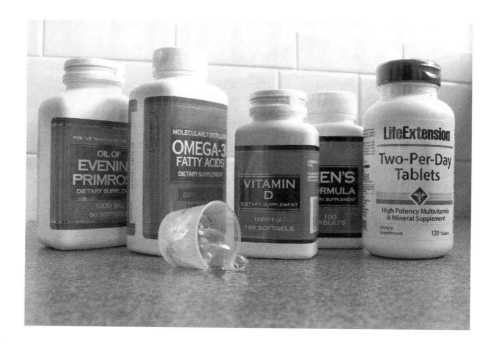

Taking Vitamins

Your Decision Rests on Several Ideas

Think about these concepts:

- Your metabolism, operating on 100,000 year-old genetic systems, is not experiencing all the nutrition that genes are expecting, so your immune and repair systems may not be working at their best.

- Your system may have some more modern metabolic needs than a "usual diet" can meet.

- Your own taste preferences may mean you don't eat certain foods so you are missing some key nutrients in your daily intake. Are you eating ½ cup of beans every day, or fish three times a week?

I would suggest that you ask yourself whether your diet as you eat now is as nourishing as your system really needs it to be?

Vitamins are a great insurance policy for nutrient adequacy.

Should You Take a Multivitamin? Yes. ————

Think about taking a better than average vitamin each day, to cover some key nutrients. The term "multivitamin" has no special meaning. There is no standard for the composition. Many stores have their generic bottles of multivitamins. Drug companies make them too, like Centrum from Glaxo, and Theragran-M from Bristol Myers Squibb. They can contain any amount of vitamin E, or vitamin C in a pill. They may or may not include minerals like magnesium and selenium. Again, there is no prescribed amount of vitamins or minerals that a supplement must contain. You need to check to see if the amount you need is provided.

Vitamin and Mineral Checklist

NUTRIENT	SAFE AND USEFUL DOSE
Vitamin C	250 mg (milligrams) on up to 1000 mg
Vitamin D	1,000 iu (international units) minimum, 2,000 iu better
	Many people find they need 4,000 iu per day.
Vitamin E	100 iu up to 400 iu, but at 200 iu or higher, get "mixed tocopherols"
B-complex vitamins	which is B-1, B-2, B-6, B-12 all blended together, as B-complex 25, or B-complex 50. In the B-complex, ideally vitamin B9 comes as folate, not folic acid.
Magnesium	100 mg on up to 400 mg
Selenium	100 mcg (micrograms) on up to 200 mcg
Chromium	200 mcg

Your Multivitamin
Some Key Nutrient Levels to Aim For

In the chart on the previous page are useful ranges of some key vitamins and minerals to look for in a multivitamin multi-mineral supplement. There should be 50% to 100% of the daily value for all possible nutrients, like copper, boron, manganese, but you will want higher quantities of certain Paleo era nutrients.

Useful lower levels of intervention are listed here, and safe upper levels of usefulness are also shown. It can still happen that in some special cases, even higher amounts of items like vitamin C or vitamin B6 or other agents may be useful for conditions like shingles or carpal tunnel syndrome, but those therapies are for a limited time.

I like to keep it all uncomplicated and efficient. You don't need to be buying 7 bottles of vitamins. As of this 2018 printing, here are a few useful products that are available nationally, that come close to this expert blend.

Examples of enhanced multivitamins

ITEM	AVAILABLE AT
50+ Men Supernutrition	Whole Foods
50+ Women Supernutrition	Whole Foods
Active Senior Multivitamins by Rainbow Light	Vitamin Shoppe
Two-Per-Day Tablets by Life Extension	Vitamin Shoppe
Active 50+ Once Daily Multivitamin & Minerals	Trader Joe's

Enhanced Multivitamins: 100% RDA for usual vitamins, 100 mg Magnesium, 100 mcg Selenium, plus approx. 10 X RDA B-complex, vitamin C & vitamin E.

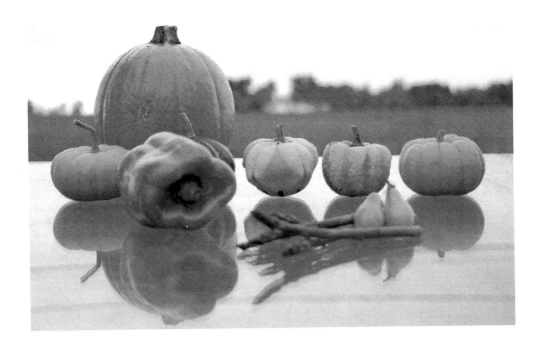

OK, so you have been reading a lot about eating well. How is your diet right now?

The following work sheet can help you decide if you're truly eating as well as you need to.

Quick Diet Screening

Date: _____

When eating your daily meals, what assortment of foods do you have?

Check off all foods you ate today.

BREAKFAST

Protein:	❏ eggs	❏ cheese	❏ cottage cheese
	❏ ham	❏ steak	❏ whey protein powder
Grain/starch:	❏ bagel	❏ cereal	❏ donut	❏ grits
	❏ muffin	❏ pancake	❏ pizza	❏ toast
	❏ waffle			
Dairy:	❏ cheese	❏ cocoa	❏ milk	❏ soy milk
	❏ yogurt			
Fruit:	❏ apple	❏ banana	❏ grapefruit	❏ peach
	❏ pineapple	❏ raisins	❏ watermelon	
Juice:	❏ cranberry	❏ orange	❏ pineapple	

LUNCH

Protein:	❏ cheese	❏ chicken	❏ ham	❏ hamburger
	❏ turkey			
Grain/starch:	❏ beans	❏ bread	❏ pasta	❏ rice
	❏ tortilla	❏ sub roll		
Vegetables:	❏ broccoli	❏ carrots	❏ celery	❏ salad greens
	❏ tomato			
Beverage:	❏ beer	❏ coffee	❏ juice	❏ milk
	❏ tea	❏ diet soda	❏ regular soda	
Dessert:	❏ cake	❏ candy bar	❏ cookies	❏ ice cream
	❏ pie			

SNACK

- ❏ cake
- ❏ candy
- ❏ chocolate
- ❏ cookies
- ❏ crackers
- ❏ fruit
- ❏ ice cream
- ❏ nuts/seeds
- ❏ pie
- ❏ pizza
- ❏ pretzels
- ❏ yogurt
- ❏ coffee
- ❏ iced tea
- ❏ milk
- ❏ diet soda
- ❏ regular soda

DINNER

Protein:	❏ beef	❏ burgers	❏ chicken	❏ fish
	❏ lamb	❏ pizza	❏ pork	❏ turkey
Starch/grain:	❏ beans/frijoles		❏ arroz/corn	❏ pasta
	❏ platano	❏ rice	❏ tortilla	
Vegetables:	❏ carrots	❏ broccoli	❏ greens	❏ string beans
	❏ salad	❏ tomato		
Oil:	❏ butter	❏ corn oil	❏ fried food	❏ gravy
	❏ margarine	❏ olive oil	❏ sour cream	
Dessert:	❏ cake	❏ cookies	❏ ice cream	❏ pie

EVENING SNACKS

Beverage:	❏ juice	❏ diet soda	❏ regular soda	
	❏ beer	❏ wine		
Grain/starch:	❏ cake	❏ chips	❏ crackers	❏ popcorn
	❏ pretzels			
Fruit:	❏ apple	❏ apricots	❏ banana	❏ berries
	❏ melon	❏ orange		
Protein:	❏ cheese	❏ cold cuts	❏ hot dog	❏ pepperoni

Look at the foods you checked.

Are you eating enough servings for each group each day?

3 Proteins	1 - 2 Dairy/calcium foods
3 Fruits	2 Vegetables
1 Legume	1 Nuts or Seeds

PART 5:

Nourishing Your Body Parts

The next sections of this book present a head to toe review of body parts and systems that may benefit from medical nutrition therapy as people age. Food and supplement therapies for slowing aging or restoring body systems to good function are presented in detail.

Being very well nourished might slow the aging process, and could reduce the need for medications.

Many people over the age of 50 have some body parts that are not working optimally. It may be higher blood pressure, or some finicky bowels, or acid indigestion. Cholesterol and triglycerides counts can be too high. Crohn's disease, Ulcerative Colitis, and Multiple Sclerosis may start to feel worse too. A doctor may prescribe a number of medicines to manage these conditions, and very often people find the number of pills they take keeps rising, as do the number of side effects. People take all sorts of pills, but don't feel all that healthier. People taking prescription medicines are frequently not happy about being on them. Little wonder that non-compliance with even filling prescriptions is as high as 31%.[81]

The idea here is to try a smart program of diet plus some added vitamins, minerals or other nutritional items to help cells function well.

The previous sections of this book have been about helping you eat the healthiest food plan, as we know it. They explain why you want to be taking a better than average multivitamin.

The next sections are to help you focus on areas of special interest to you, your friends, and your family. The discussion is more technical. You may not understand all the details, but you at least get the concept that diet and added nutrient supplements can improve your wellbeing.

You might already have the sense that nutrition can help you function better and decrease your dependence on medicines that simply manage your symptoms. Now, your project is to learn the details of what will repair the essential systems in you. You can take this book and consult with a savvy nutrition professional for help. Email the author if you have questions. As you have likely noticed, there are dozens of references in well-known scientific journals supporting the suggestions here.

Feed Your Head _____

Brain Cell Support

Slowing or reversing the general aging process in the brain is on many people's minds. Here is a quick **science lesson**. The brain is composed of many nerve cells that must talk to each other. One cell communicates with another through a chemical messenger called a "neurotransmitter." The nutrition fundamentals are that a cell must make the neurotransmitter in adequate amounts for a good signal to happen. Also, the cell on the receiving end must be in decent shape in order to pick up the message. Nutrients that support production of neurotransmitters, and that compose the receptor cell surface are the focus here.

Brain signal strength matters to all body systems. Some signals regulate moods or ability to sleep. Other signals help memory. Good serotonin flow contributes to your getting a good nights sleep and your avoiding depression. Other signals help memory. Still others help blood sugar regulation, and digestion. The heart's response to both physical and mental stress depends on brain signals. If your brain is not at its best, the rest of you won't be either.

Perhaps you have encountered people who seem cranky and difficult in older age. It can be easy to judge them as grouchy personalities who simply lack a loving perspective on people and events. However, there can be a big biological explanation for their attitude and behavior. Some people with Alzheimer's are experiencing memory loss while others experience anxiety and have more aggressive behavior. It is a change in cell architecture that is likely the cause. Remember, the building blocks of brain cells are groceries.

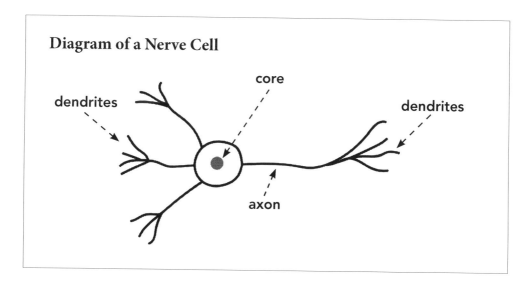

Diagram of a Nerve Cell

core

dendrites

dendrites

axon

Too Many Free Radicals Can Be One Component of Aging in the Brain.

Many of the nutrients discussed as key components of the Paleolithic Diet are vital to brain cell health.[82] You have heard that "fish is brain food." Cell membranes are made up of a blend of proteins, cholesterol and fats. Well, when more of the fat in the brain cell walls is the omega-3 EPA/DHA type, the brain works better. Data from the Framingham Heart Study has shown that people consuming fish three times a week, and therefore having higher DHA levels in their blood and brain, cut their risk of senile dementia in half![83] Remember, there is no drug to reverse dementia.

Let food be your first medicine.
Try a therapeutic food and nutrient program to manage your ailments.
After improving nutrition, the need for medicines frequently drops.

How many people truly eat fish 3 times a week? Government research data says 50% of the population eats zero ounces of fish a week. A bit fewer than 10% of the people in this country eat 8 ounces of fish a week. For reasons of cost, convenience or taste, many people are not consuming much fish, especially the kind that provides EPA/DHA fats. As mentioned before, researchers like Colonel Hibbeln, a brilliant physician in the U.S. Public Health Service, would declare poor brain function to be not a sign of disease, but a sign of malnutrition over time.[84] The nutrient lacking is omega-3 fish oil: EPA/DHA.

Taking omega-3, EPA/DHA fish oil pills is an important consideration for vegetarians and people who don't eat fish at all. Technically, getting 0.6 to 1.2% of total calories as omega-3 is the goal.[85] If you live on 2200 calories a day, then 1% is 20 calories. There are 9 calories per gram of fat, which suggests that you need to get 2 grams fish oil per day to keep your brain in good shape. Most fish oil pills are about 1,000mg which is 1 gram. The specific part of the fish oil that most helps the brain is the EPA/DHA part of the 1,000mg pill. If you get into more scientific detail, you can check the amount of EPA/DHA you are getting in your pills. The nutrient label on the pills lists how many pills it takes of a particular brand, to get enough EPA and DHA.

This is a sample label from a Nordic Naturals Ultimate omega-3 Fish Oils product.

Notice the data is for **2 pills**, not one. You can see how much EPA and how much DHA the two pills have in total. The total omega-3's part of the label can include some omega-3 that is not EPA/DHA and does not have the biological activity that you want. Pay attention to the EPA/DHA numbers. You want 500mg per day or more.

Serving Size	2 SOFTGELS
Servings Per Container	30
Amount Per Serving	
CALORIES	18
CALORIES FROM FAT	18
TOTAL FAT	2 gm
SATURATED FAT	0 gm
TRANS FAT	0 gm
TOTAL OMEGA-3'S	1280 mg
EPA	650 mg
DHA	450 mg
OTHER OMEGA-3'S	180 mg

Supplementation at 500 mg/day of total EPA/DHA is wise.

For people who know they have heart disease, getting a total of 1,000 mg per day of EPA/DHA is a good idea.[86] People who are lacto-ovo vegetarians are consuming the plant form of omega-3 fat called ALA, which gives them some cardio protection, but are missing the vital brain support of EPA/DHA. The amount of ALA that the body converts to the brain-active forms EPA and DHA is a function of what types of, and what total volume of, fats are in the diet. I am worried that vegetarians consume inadequate amounts of DHA so less will be available for best brain function. Others share this concern.[87] While not making an official recommendation to take supplements, Drs. Johnson and Schaeffer, in mentioning their Framingham Heart Study research data, point out that an average fish oil pill will usually have at least the 180 mg of DHA, the amount to consume daily, to replicate the amount received in the 2.7 servings per week fish intake that lowered the risk of senile dementia.[88]

You may need to take 2 to 3 fish oil pills a day to get 500mg of EPA/DHA.

Size Matters: Foods For Thought

As people age, their brains are vulnerable to some shrinkage. There is a familiar phrase, "Size matters." This is especially true for brains. Brain size is related to thinking capacity; a smaller brain is not as good at processing thoughts.

The brain gets smaller from losing its battle with stray electrons (free radicals).[89] Stray electrons cause irritation, leading to inflammation, leading to brain cell shrinking. An easy analogy to illustrate the process: picture a grape on the vine in the sun, withering in the heat, becoming a raisin. The source of the free radicals can be any number of chronic illnesses, like arthritis. An interesting fact is that carrying excess abdominal area (visceral) fat turns out to cause inflammation that can cause brain shrinking in middle-aged adults.[90] Given the number of overweight and obese people in America, the potential incidence of people with dementia is staggering. Achieving and maintaining a trim, fit weight is challenging, but if you are worried about memory loss in older age, reducing belly-area fat removes one risk you can do something about. Again, this is not an easy task, as many people know.

The Mediterranean Diet, coupled with routine exercise, lowers the risk of Alzheimer's more than either diet or exercise can individually accomplish.[91]

A fundamental aspect of Alzheimer's is inflammation, modulated by the chemical messenger substance (cytokine) called Tumor Necrosis Factor alpha (TNFa). Alzheimer's is a bigger risk for people with other inflammatory conditions. So not only would you say, "Size matters," you can add, "Stray electrons matter" too. An example: accelerated rates of brain shrinking are happening in "healthy middle-aged" people with metabolic syndrome, even without diabetes.[92] (Metabolic syndrome is the presence of some extra sugar and fat in the blood, plus slightly elevated blood pressure.)

In Alzheimer's, brain neuron function is disrupted by free radicals and by the presence of a plaque called Amyloid-beta. How does the plaque land there? One simplified explanation is that when a bit of magnesium is replaced with a bit of calcium in brain cell structures, Amyloid toxicity happens.[93][94] Much research is happening around how or why this occurs, and how other nutrients, like zinc and copper can disrupt the process.[95] Remember, more than half the country has a diet with inadequate amounts of zinc.

Many factors play a role in the number and fate of free radicals irritating and shrinking brain cells. Foremost, the amount of antioxidant capacity in the diet affects how the brain copes with the stray electrons generated by everyday metabolism. Nutrition advice for reducing risk the of senility and Alzheimer's starts with the food plan already outlined here. Omega-3 EPA/DHA fats are anti-inflammatory, and do lower TNFa levels in people directly. When obese people lose weight, their TNFa levels drop as well.

Here are a few food ideas to accent in your diet. Follow the advice of David Heber, MD PhD, in his book: What Color Is Your Diet? All the colors of the fruit and vegetables in the diet are various wavelengths of antioxidant action. Other substances, known as phytochemicals, in foods like dark chocolate, acai berries, red grape skins and red wine also have free-radical squelching properties. The kinds of fats in the diet also play a role in brain cell function. You know about fish oils. Olive oil is also anti-inflammatory. Replacing some grain calories with some olive oil calories seems to be one of the healthy elements of the Mediterranean diet.

Berries For The Brain

Some new research reports from the USDA Aging Center in Boston and other groups are exciting. Supplementing the diets of laboratory animals, and then of aged people, with one half cup of blueberries,[96] and other foods, like strawberries, almonds or Concord grapes, improves memory function in as little as 12 weeks![97] This change in memory in just three month's time is astounding.

I already mentioned magnificent magnesium a few pages back. Here is yet another reason to pay attention to magnesium: its value in supporting brain cells. Magnesium as a food mineral plays a role in over 100 body chemistry reactions: brain cell construction and function included. Much of magnesium's activity helps squelch free radicals and thereby reduces inflammation.[98] Remember, magnesium is a nutrient under-consumed the by the US population, especially older people. The same goes for zinc. Like magnesium, zinc supports systems that repair proteins and squelch inflammation, especially in the nervous system.[99] So be sure the multivitamin/mineral pill you take includes at least 100mg of magnesium and 15mg of zinc.

Check Your Homocysteine Levels for Brain Not Just Heart Health

A vitamin supplement for coronary artery support could be important for another reason. Homocysteine (HCYS) and methylmalonic acid (MMA) are substances that irritate the brain and are part of the aging process. When blood levels of HCYS and MMA are higher than ideal, it is usually a sign that B-vitamins are running low. A small study of several hundred older people, who had normal B-complex vitamin levels in their blood, showed that they still had elevated numbers for HCYS and MMA. When given a supplement containing: 1mg vitamin B12, 1 mg Folic Acid, and 5 mg vitamin B6, their elevated numbers dropped to normal in about ¾ of cases in just 5 to 12 days.[100] These supplement amounts are not much different than those included in common "Stress Tab" B-complex vitamins sold in pharmacies across the country.

The above study brings up the issue of how to test for vitamin deficiency. Determining "normal" blood tests for vitamin B -12 are a controversy. Are blood levels truly a good indicator?[101] Another aspect is whether the current RDA for people over 50 needs some adjusting. While those debates lumber along, what you want to be looking at is the simple fact, outlined in the publically available article: *Homocysteine-lowering by B vitamins slows the rate of accelerated brain atrophy in mild cognitive impairment: a randomized controlled trial.*[102] Various studies place the number of people with low vitamin B -12 levels at a minimum of 15% of the population. Others suggest the number may be higher for people taking medicines that reduce stomach acid production. The acid reflux treatment drug Omeprazole can reduce B12 absorption by 66% or more, depending on dose.[103] Some people monitor Homocysteine for concerns about cardiac health. Watching homocysteine for brain wellness is a far bigger reason.

Instead of relying on some variable blood tests for B-vitamin levels, what could you do? This all comes down to the idea that taking a Stress Tab level of B-complex vitamins (3 to 5 times the RDA) is a good brain health maintenance move, with no risk of adverse events. The multivitamins previously listed here will have this extra amount of B-complex vitamins included, so no need to shop for a second pill.

One other aspect of brain chemistry and mood I want to point out is that depression is not just about serotonin levels, as is commonly believed. Taking drugs like Prozac or Seroquil are not a solid fix. In his book: *Talking Back To Prozac: What Doctors Aren't Telling You About Today's Most Controversial Drug,* Peter Breggin, MD mentions that thousands of people dropped out of Prozac

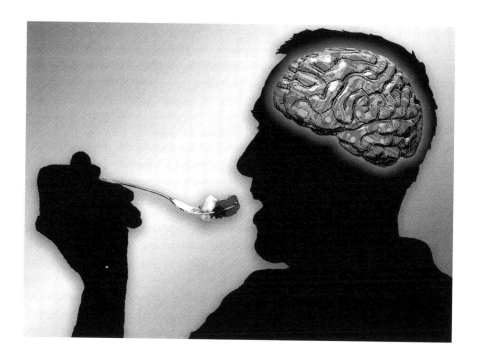

drug studies due to side effects, so that the FDA ended up approving Prozac for the treatment of depression, using data on from fewer than 300 people, who were treated for just 6 weeks. At best, about 10-20 % of people experience benefit from Selective Serotonin Reuptake Inhibitor (SSRI) drugs. A recent paper reviewing all antidepressant drug trials commented that data is scant: few numbers, and weak associations. The authors commented that side effects are significant, and doctors should be cautious prescribing SSRI's.[104] For serotonin drug therapy, one German journal says a placebo is as effective as the real medicine.[105] There are other events at work in the brains of people with depression and anxiety. A complex interplay of chemicals, inflammation, and blend of neurotransmitters is likely operative. [106 107 108]

I hate to sound dark and dismal, but here goes. As the population ages, and the percent of obese people rises, the horde of brain-challenged people will be staggering. How society and the medical system will cope with the unprecedented numbers of senile people is unknown. The dollar cost alone will be alarming. Don't get caught up in the tidal wave. It won't be fun or pretty being in the flotilla. Look at food, fitness and supplements as your best hedge against a future with a dim brain. You are what you shop for!

Brain Cells and Brain Circuitry

Brain cell "plasticity" is a new idea that is getting a lot of attention. It is about preserving brain function through mind-body exercises. Learning a musical instrument is one of the best activities for this, as it involves conceptualizing thoughts, and coordinating muscles. The brain has to open up new passageways to make all this happen. This means growing new cellular links. Up until recently, no one thought nerve cells could grow.[109] Herbert Benson, MD, the champion of mind-body medicine and The Relaxation Response, currently at Massachusetts General Hospital in Boston, has stunning new data on using guided imagery and meditation to repair damaged nerve cells.[110] Benson's research is showing that you may be able to think your way back to better health.

The Emerging Revolution In Health:
Energy Medicine, Even for Brain

Is life all about Newton's laws of motion and attraction? Your smart science brain says that sophisticated chemical reactions run the world. You also know that genes are a big part of your medical fate. But wait, kids adopted into families get cancer at the same rate as the new family, not at the rate of the family they came from. So maybe they eat the same food, and have the same lifestyle. How about the case of a wife who sends loving and nurturing thoughts to her sick husband, who is sealed in a 2000 lb. metal box, and his heart rate and blood pressure change? No chemicals involved here. One other idea: you sometimes walk into a room full of people and say to yourself, "I don't like the feel of this room." We might say that your sixth sense is picking up on something. What we all know is that thoughts exist, and they can have physiological consequences, like fear raising pulse and blood pressure. What science cannot yet tell you is how a thought happens. It may result in a change in chemical events, but a thought is more than just chemical action. Birds fly in formation, and make moves in sequence that are faster than chemistry itself. So there are energy events that we see occurring, but chemistry alone, and therefore nutrition, cannot explain them. Enter Albert Einstein, and the world of quantum physics and quantum entanglement.

New Age physics is on the verge of helping you stay healthy or repair old damage. I would like to direct you to an amazing documentary film, from 2010, *The Living Matrix – The Science of Healing*. You can go to a web site: www.documentaryaddict.com to view it. It presents exciting news about coming advances in healing. A number of physicists and medical doctors explain the limits of biological healing. They explain the world of energy medicine, and how it can contribute to the healing of chronic illness. Bruce Lipton, MD, PhD, is also a compelling author, and research scientist. His book, *The Biology of Belief* describes how the mind could be instrumental in directing biological repair. I mention the book and the movie because we are trained to think of the realms of Chi (an Eastern concept of energy) and yoga and such as to be woo-woo, that is, outlandishly unscientific . Here are some of the brightest, most scientifically credentialed people on the planet, laying out the cutting edge science in the realm of healing. Take advantage of it! I explain more of this in the Tong Ren energy healing section.

The heart is a very sensitive muscle;
its cells damage quickly and easily.

Cholesterol and Cardiovascular Disease _____

The heart, arteries and veins form the cardiovascular system. In one sense, the system is simply a pump and the set of pipes that carry blood, oxygen, nutrients and debris to and from all parts of the body. Arteries and veins are talented; they flex, expand and contract on demand, depending on the need for more circulation to certain places in a hurry. If pipes corrode internally, flow is diminished. In aging, the system also loses its ability to be as flexible as needed. You may have heard the term, "hardening of the arteries." As you can imagine, the basic flow and flexibility properties decline when hardening happens.

A plaque containing calcium and cholesterol constitutes the corrosive material in walls of the arteries. Simply put, the interior diameter of the pipes becomes smaller which reduces flow capacity. With the plaque there, the endothelium (the cells lining the arteries) doesn't function correctly. For instance, the arterial walls may not let cholesterol pass through them so well, out of the blood and on into cells. They may accidently contract, when they were supposed to relax: which is something called "endothelial dysfunction". When the very fine blood vessels of the heart become corroded, the cardiac cells are at risk for lack of oxygen. When a bit of plaque breaks off some artery wall and blocks an artery servicing the heart, you get a heart attack. Muscle (heart) deprived of oxygen is horribly painful, and also dies rapidly. With age and other stresses, like free radical damage, the cardiovascular system can become corroded.

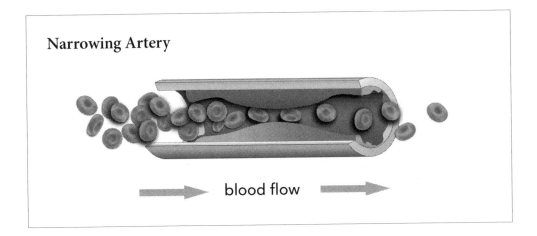

Narrowing Artery

blood flow

How Arteries Corrode, and the Consequences

In the diagram below you see an artery. Notice the artery has cells on the inner lining and has a muscle layer. There are pores in the lining. When something like "oxidized cholesterol" (cholesterol made sticky by stray electrons) falls into a pore, it festers, and immune CD36 cells come to bat clean up. There is an inflammatory response for awhile and though things all settle down after the clean up, there is a small scar left. The analogy is much like an acne pimple. Something gets in a skin pore, some inflammation happens, and a small scar remains. The accumulated scars form the plaque in arterial walls.

Let me repeat: what gets into the cracks and causes the trouble are bits of "oxidized cholesterol". This is cholesterol that itself has been a bit nicked and scratched up by stray electrons in the blood stream. Stray electrons are the same agents that rust tin cans and car bumpers. They are electrons that fell out of their original orbit, likely at some chemical reaction elsewhere in the body. Antioxidants, like vitamin C and vitamin E and the colors in fruits and vegetables can capture stray electrons. You hear about the properties of red wine and dark chocolate doing the same free radical scavenging. In the past few years, there is a renewed emphasis on what is the real issue for heart disease prevention. More experts are encouraging people to eat more foods that scavenge for stray electrons. They see this as the real way to avoid getting heart disease.

While learning advice about how to lower cholesterol, you need to know that having a lower cholesterol number is not the whole story for avoiding or treating heart disease. There is the French paradox. People in that country (and Switzerland) have generally higher cholesterol numbers than Americans do but they don't have as much heart disease. Many factors could account for their better vascular health including a less stressful culture. One area of significant interest is the antioxidant value of their total diet, including the red grape/red wine antioxidant compound called Resveratrol they consume. In a sense, it is not the presence of cholesterol that matters but how much "oxidized cholesterol" is around.

Cholesterol Numbers
Different for People Over Age 50 or 60

A quick review of what cholesterol numbers mean.

Total Cholesterol in the blood reflects 3 component parts.

- **LDL-cholesterol**, the potentially sticky stuff that can clog arteries.

- **HDL cholesterol**, the cholesterol that is in a package on the way to the trash.

- **Triglyceride fat**, which is fuel fat molecules that travel the bloodstream with a cholesterol wrapper.

Combine LDL, plus HDL, plus 20% of the Triglyceride value and you get the total Cholesterol number which you see on your lab reports from your medical office.

It seems that very high cholesterol numbers contribute to premature heart disease but in the Framingham Heart Study data, somewhat elevated cholesterol is connected to all causes of mortality mostly at age 40, and not at all by age 80. Higher cholesterol levels mostly connect to **heart disease mortality** at ages 40, 50 and 60. In an article in the Archives of Internal Medicine, the authors point out **that lower cholesterol** is associated with **higher non-heart mortality after age 50**, and that physicians should be cautious about initiating cholesterol-lowering treatment in men and women above 65 to 70 years of age until trials show efficacy or cost effectiveness.[111]

A group at Yale also pointed out that in people over age 70, there was no significant association between blood cholesterol levels and either coronary artery or all causes of mortality.[112] Again, I will point out that lifestyle elements, particularly diet quality and fitness level, are far more predictive of health risk.

Lower cholesterol numbers are associated with higher mortality in some studies. A Honolulu research group, based on data from 3,527 Japanese-American men age 71 to 93, observed for 20 years, says:

> *These data cast doubt on the scientific justification for lowering [total] cholesterol to very low concentrations (<4.65 mmol/L =180mg/dL) in elderly people.*[113]

Famous drug treatment studies to lower cardiac morbidity and mortality like the Helsinki Heart Study did reduce cardiac issues, but did not extend total life expectancy. Interestingly, the incidence of violent death (accident or suicide) incidence rose.[114]

Can Cholesterol Be Too Low?
Less than 181mg/dL *or* less than 160mg/dL?

A broad survey of healthy rural Japanese men and women age 40 to 69, found that over the course of 12 years, very low cholesterol, less than 160mg/dL (< 4.14 mmol/L) was associated with a greater incidence of heart failure, stroke and cancer fatalities than moderate range 160 – 200 mg/dL (4.14 – 5.17mmol/L) numbers.[115] (For people wanting a statistic: the hazard ratio was 1.49 in men, and 1.5 for women.)

An Israeli study watching 4,000 people also found that people who were most compliant with their statin drug, and got their LDL cholesterol to below 70mg/dL, had no extra benefit when compared to compliant people who just got their LDL cholesterol to the 70 to 100 range. Interestingly, among people who were about 50% compliant with taking their statin, a cholesterol below 70 was better than being in the 70 to 100 range.[116] This suggests that some people are more sensitive to the cholesterol-lowering effects of statins, and that less drug exposure plays out ok. What it says, too, is that driving peoples' cholesterol numbers down with even higher drug exposure is not particularly beneficial. One last point in this regard, in older people with coronary artery disease, a low total cholesterol, about 160 to 180, is beneficial, but in people with heart failure without arterial disease, higher cholesterol numbers, like 200 to 220, produce better outcomes.[117] The bottom line is that if you have some second thoughts about taking a statin for **preventing** heart trouble, there is no solid data that shows you will be better off with the medicine; and a not insignificant amount of research says you should be careful about taking one.[118]

The Fed's Guidelines for Your Cholesterol

The National Cholesterol Education Program (NCEP) guidelines, created at the National Institute of Health (NIH), say total cholesterol should be < 200 mg, Triglycerides be < 150 mg, and HDL be > 40 mg for men and > 45 mg for women. LDL (sticky) cholesterol should be < 99 mg, or < 130 mg or < 160 mg, depending on age and other events in a person's health. There is much controversy over these guidelines, in part because people with significant ties to the pharmaceutical industry are the ones who set the standards.

Cholesterol by the numbers

TOTAL CHOLESTEROL	MMOL/LITER OF BLOOD		MG/DL
Ideal Total Cholesterol	< 5.13 mmol/L of blood	=	< 200 mg/dL
Borderline high	5.13 - 6.13	=	200 to 220
High	>6.13 mmol/L	=	> 220

A 2004 letter sent to the head of the NIH, the National Heart Lung Blood Institute, and NCEP directors, signed by many prominent physicians, and professors from Harvard University, The University of Michigan, Stanford University, and Tufts Medical School, and endorsed by Senators Edward Kennedy (MA), Judd Greg (NH), Joseph Lieberman (CT), Henry Waxman (CA) and others wrote:

> In petitioning for an independent review, we are not arguing that statins are not helpful for many people with elevated risk of heart disease. However, there is strong evidence to suggest that an objective, independent re-evaluation of the scientific evidence from the five new studies of statin therapy would lead to different conclusions than those presented by the current NCEP. ….

While the latest 2013 NCEP report, like the 2001 guidelines before it, notes that lifestyle modification should be a first line of therapy to prevent heart disease, the sad fact is that these recommendations are being largely ignored, partly because the "experts," many of whom have conflicts of interest through their relationships with statin manufacturers, focus ever more attention on lowering cholesterol with expensive drugs. The vast majority of heart disease can be prevented by adopting healthy habits.

The American people are poorly served when government-sanctioned clinical recommendations, uncritically amplified by the media, misdirect attention and resources to expensive medical therapies that may not be scientifically justified.[119]

The 2013, cholesterol treatment guidelines are also controversial, as even more apparently healthy people are directed to take a statin drug. A November 17, 2013 article in *The New York Times* has the headline: **Risk Calculator For Cholesterol Appears Flawed**, and quotes Harvard Medical School cardiologist Dr. Paul M. Ridker and biostatistics expert Dr. Nancy Cook.

If you have a heart disease diagnosis, you most likely need to be on some dose of a statin drug. The effectiveness of this drug may be less likely about its making your cholesterol count low, and more likely about reducing inflammation in your arteries. There is always the issue of side effects and some scientists urge avoiding high dose statins in most cases, due to worries about liver and muscle damage.

Without a heart disease diagnosis, a diet that gets your cholesterol numbers somewhat lower has many total body health benefits. Medicines that get you to these low numbers may not be of any benefit, and may actually have unwanted side effects.

Dariush Mozaffarian, MD, Ph D. (Dean of the Tufts University Friedman School of Nutrition Science & Policy, and the Jean Mayer Chair and Professor of Nutrition), a board-certified cardiologist and PhD epidemiologist, is on an international committee that looks at Nutrition and Global Burden of Chronic Disease. Starting back in 2005, he was publishing information pointing out that beef consumption and saturated fat intake were less connected to heart disease than previously thought.[120] In recent years, he's been even more emphatic that eating adequate amounts of fruits and vegetables, rather than avoiding saturated fat, is the way to heart health and prevention of cardiovascular disease.[121] If you have some time, watch his lecture at a Harvard Medical School symposium on how it is actually the lack of fruits and vegetables that is a primary risk factor for the development of heart disease.[122] A good study that proves this point comes out of Lyon, France.

The Lyon Heart Study

Diet has a huge impact on blood supply to the heart. In Lyon, France, researchers asked 600 people who were in the hospital after having had a heart attack to go on a diet, to see if it could prevent their returning to the hospital with another heart attack. They placed 300 people on the NCEP1 diet (The National Cholesterol Education Program) asking them to eat a low fat, low cholesterol diet. They were to avoid eggs, and have just small servings of meat, chicken or fish. They were encouraged to eat more pasta, bagels and cereal: essentially the advice of the first Food Guide Pyramid. The other 300 people were asked to follow the diet eaten by the people on the island of Crete, near Greece.

This island has a very low incidence of heart disease. People consume more fish, seafood, legumes, salads, fruits, nuts and seeds. The Cretan diet has more carbohydrates from fruits and beans and less from grains than the NCEP diet. It allows more milligrams of cholesterol per day. It also has more fat grams per day than the NCEP plan, but the fats are from olive oil, a mono-unsaturated fat.

After 27 months, they checked to see how people were doing. Well, both groups had nice lower cholesterol and triglyceride numbers, and healthy HDL levels. However heart attack rates were radically different.

There were 33 heart attacks on the NCEP plan:
16 fatal, 17 non-fatal.

There were 8 heart attacks on the Crete plan:
3 fatal, 5 non fatal.

Let me say this again so you really understand these results. Even in the setting of nice cholesterol numbers, there was a 76% drop in death rate by eating a better diet. Cholesterol numbers were fine on both types of diets. **Food made the difference**. No prescription drug is potent enough to achieve these outcomes.

The study continued. After 48 months, the **cardiac death rate was still 56%** lower on the Crete food plan and there was a **61% drop in cancer death rates!**[123]

The science concept here is that on a food plan with healthy fats and more antioxidant foods, your arteries stay less inflamed, and blood vessels stay more flexible. It seems that immune system cells work better too. Imagine, grilled shrimp on a mixed green salad, with some cannellini beans in it for lunch, plus a snack of walnuts and grapes a little later, or almonds and apricots. Sounds like a tolerable lunch to me.

More studies are showing up that point out that the development of heart disease is not so much about avoiding dietary saturated fat and cholesterol, but consuming enough antioxidant foods such as fruits and vegetables. Information from what 84,000 nurses are eating also attests to the idea that having more vegetables, especially leafy green ones, plus vitamin C-rich fruits in the diet reduces risk of heart disease.[124]

If people do not have enough anti-inflammation compounds in their body, then their plumbing corrodes.

There are risk factors besides diet that raise the chance you'll get heart disease. These conditions all have an inflammation component:

- Smoking
- Obesity
- Hypertension
- Diabetes

Having high total cholesterol and a high LDL is a factor in premature heart disease, but after age 60, it may not be so important.[125] For someone age 55 or 60 and older, it is time to be rethinking cholesterol numbers, and health status.

A Science Lesson
"Relative" Versus "Absolute" Risk Reduction in Clinical Trials

Below are some numbers you might see as results in a clinical trial for heart attack prevention with a cholesterol-lowering drug. There is usually a placebo group (also labeled the "placebo arm" of a trial, then the drug treatment group or arm. Let's say the trial lasted 2 years.

Example results from a clinical trial

	PEOPLE TREATED	HEART ATTACKS
Placebo arm	1,000	40
Treatment arm	1,000	20

You can assess the benefit of the trial in two ways. There is a *50% relative reduction in events*. There is also a *2% absolute risk reduction*.

> The heart attack incidence goes from 40 to 20, so a company says this is a 50% reduction in heart attack events. True, taking the study drug meant the rate of people getting heart attacks went down 50%.

> However 40 events per 1000 is a 4% heart attack rate in the placebo arm, and going down to 20 events per thousand is now a 2% rate in the treatment arm ... so you can see that taking the study drug helped just 20 people in a thousand: it helped 2% who took it. This sounds different than it being a 50% reduction in heart attacks, doesn't it? These numbers represent an example of relative versus absolute risk reduction in science reporting.

Another Science Lesson
Number Needed to Treat in Clinical Trials

In the above example you can see that 20 people benefited out of the 1000 people given a study drug. This is the same as saying 10 people for every 500 treated or 1 person for every 50 people. The term "number needed to treat" refers to the calculation of how many people will have to take a drug, for one person to receive benefit. Here the "number needed to treat" is 50. As you read the next section, you will now have a better understanding of what Dr. Abramson is saying.

There is an incredibly informative book: *Overdosed America: The Broken Promise Of American Medicine*, written by John Abramson, MD.[126] He reports the deception used in published clinical trials that get reported in medical journal articles. He explains the difference between changes in "relative risk" versus "absolute risk" in trial results. Here is an example he gives. In the West Of Scotland Coronary Prevention Study (WOSCOPS), half of the 6,000 men in the study were given the statin drug Pravocol, 40 mg a day. These men had an average LDL of 192, and 44% of them smoked cigarettes. Of the guys on Pravocol, there was a 31% reduction in 'relative risk' of having a heart attack. This sounds great, but the 'actual risk' was much lower. As he says, "100 people would have to take Pravocol for 2 years to prevent a single heart attack. In order to prevent a single death, 100 men in the WOSCOPS study would have to take Pravocol for 5½ years." OK, if you have a cholesterol level at 220, and your doctor suggests you take a pill to be healthier, would you take the drug, knowing that you have a one in 100 chance of benefiting from it in the next 2 to 5 years?

I worked at the Harvard University Student-Faculty Health Service for many years. I attended many social receptions that featured fruit platters, along with cheese and cracker plates. One day, a doc and I were next to the cheese platter, and he said to me, "I suppose you don't eat this stuff," as he popped a few cubes of cheddar in his mouth. I replied that I am modest with my cheese consumption, due to the saturated fat content. He said, "Oh, I am not worried, I am taking Lipitor," and then proceeded to munch some brie wedges.

This is a well-trained, capable physician, whose thinking reflects the general medical perception of the dynamic utility of statin drugs in preventing heart disease. I want you to know better, though. My cheese-munching Harvard doc does not comprehend how little protection his statin drug is offering him. He is not alone, in fact. Research is now showing that statin users are paying less attention to diet, and eating more fat and gaining more weight than non-users. A JAMA Internal Medicine (Journal of the American Medical Association) article included the phrase "*gluttony in the time of statins*" in its article title.[127]

The data for people who have had a heart attack and are taking a statin drug to prevent another heart attack does show benefit. However, as you just saw from the results of the Lyon Heart Study, diet is three times more useful, so don't neglect the food part.

Some people will take every possible nutrition step they can, and still have an elevated LDL. If they are reluctant to take a statin medicine, or cannot tolerate one, I don't want them to feel that they are in imminent danger without the medicine. I want them to appreciate that diet is twice as preventative of cardiac trouble compared to medication. I also want people to appreciate that exercise is also far more potent than any medicine in preventing heart attacks. See the vitamin E discussion and how it helps prevent heart troubles later in this section. Also, there are some other nutrition tricks to do.

Reversing a Low HDL Number Is Also Very Important

Away with the bad, bring in more good. Much emphasis is placed on lowering high LDL cholesterol, but a low HDL (good cholesterol) deserves attention too. HDL is emerging as an independent risk factor of heart attacks and heart disease mortality even in people 80 years old.[128] The usual lifestyle factors that promote a good HDL number are being a trim weight, being capable of cardio-fitness activity for 45 continuous minutes, and eating a good balance of carbohydrates and fats in the diet. A deficiency of the good omega 6 fat gamma linolenic acid (GLA,) along with a deficiency in omega-3, can cause a lower HDL. Some people with a low HDL that I see in my office are often eating lots of pasta, fruits, bagels and breads. I'll ask them to replace some carbohydrate calories with nuts, seeds and olive oil, and their hunger levels will go down and their HDL levels will go up 4 or 5 points.

HDL is produced in the liver, and if the liver is stressed with inadequate amounts of antioxidant materials, HDL levels will be lower.[129] After a while on a better diet, and after taking a better antioxidant vitamin, I'll add 1 or 2 nutrient supplements to improve HDL. First, I recommend 2 grams per day of Evening Primrose oil, for the GLA fat, to rule out essential fat deficiency. I may also add 2 grams a day of the amino acid N-acetylcysteine (NAC.) This improves Glutathione (antioxidant) levels in the liver. A rise of 8-10 points of HDL can happen thanks to the NAC pills.[130]

Every Possible Nutrition Step for a Healthy Heart

First, the Mediterranean (Crete) diet is what I detailed in the original food plan, back on pages 11 to 25 , when I was describing the more Paleolithic foods plan. Let me accent some key concepts here.

Key Concepts for Reducing Heart Disease Risk

1. Eat a lot of FIBER: People eating high fiber (roughage) diets have lower cholesterol and less heart disease and diabetes. Women should try to eat 25 grams of fiber per day, and men, 35 grams per day. A good foundation is 3 servings of fruit per day, and 3 cups (cooked volume) of vegetables per day, (1 cup at lunch and 2 cups at dinner). Then add one other serious fiber dose per day, consumed as either ½ cup of a bean (legume) food, or as a serious high fiber cereal. You will get 7 grams of fiber per serving in either choice.

In the Crete diet, fruits have replaced some of the grain calories in the daily diet. This has a tremendous impact on some important metabolic events in the body.

Fruits are great fiber. Many people think they have a lot of sugar, and avoid them, and have a grain item instead. This is a mistake. Just keep the fruit portion to 100 calories and you'll be fine. Fruits contain a blend of fructose and glucose, and this mixture does not require as much insulin to process it. While you may be someone who is worrying about a blood sugar number, remember it is how insulin is clearing the sugar out of the blood on into cells that matters. A grain or starch item can frequently require more insulin to process it. Since insulin has "build fat," "retain sodium" and "make hungry" messages, keeping insulin levels lower is the desired goal. Fruits consumed with some protein, seeds or nuts will digest more slowly, keeping the insulin response lower. This is what people mean when they talk about "low glycemic load" eating. The total amount of sugar consumed is a modest dose.

Fruit pulp is the most important dietary fiber in matters of heart health.

2. FRUITS: Eat 3 or 4 servings of fruit a day. Eating an apple, a banana, or a pear each day is a good start, for a dose of the cholesterol-lowering fiber called pectin. Peaches, nectarines, berries and melons are good too. Dried fruits have fiber, as do frozen and canned. One-half cup of peaches, pears or applesauce from a can constitutes a serving as well. Look at it this way, nuts and berries as snacks worked well for cave people, and will help you too.

Recommended fruits

Apples*	Grapefruit	Peaches	Watermelon
Applesauce*	Honeydew	Pears*	Dates
Apricots	Kiwis	Pineapple	Figs
Bananas*	Lychee	Plums	Raisins
Blackberries	Mangos	Pomegranate	Cran-raisins
Blueberries	Nectarines	Raspberries	
Cantaloupe	Oranges	Red grapes	
Clementines	Papaya	Strawberries	

* These fruits have more pectin, which lowers cholesterol.

Here is an important concept. Fruit pulp contains a lot of the water-soluble fiber pectin. This kind of fiber supports the growth of healthy bacteria in the intestines. These beneficial bacteria produce some small fat molecules called short-chain fatty acids; they have names like acetate, propionate, and butyrate. These small fats are fuels for keeping cells lining the large intestine in good repair. The acetate, propionate and butyrate also go off to the liver and tell it to produce less cholesterol!

Acetate, Propionate and Butyrate, small fat particles, made by friendly microbes in the gut, travel to the liver and signal it to reduce cholesterol production.

Many people are eating a low fat and low cholesterol diet, yet their lipid numbers remain elevated. One issue may be that the liver is making too much cholesterol.

How do you get the liver to produce less? Eat fruit, and have the beneficial bacteria in the gut make acetate, propionate and butyrate.[131] These fatty substances travel from gut to the liver and "down regulate" cholesterol production.

Here is a fun fact. When you have stools that look like spongy logs and they float in the toilet bowl, this is a general signal that you have a good gut flora repertoire in your intestinal ecosystem. I tell people remember: "fruit, fiber, floaters". Asking people if they have floaters makes for great cocktail party chatter.

Most people find that their stools float about 3 to 4 weeks into eating fruit more routinely. If this is not occurring, then take a "probiotic" (opposite of antibiotic) supplement.

A good probiotic supplement will be a blend of organisms with names like "Lactobacillus acidophilus, Lactobacillus plantarum, Lactobacillus rhamnosus, Bifidobacter longum, and Bifidobacter breve.

The amount of ready-to-grow organisms in a probiotic pill is labeled as "colony forming units" and a good threshold is about **5 billion** per dose.

I have seen good results from the product **JarroDophilus EPS, 25 bil. CFU, 1 pill per day.**

3. VEGETABLES: Eating at least 2 to 3 cups per day of vegetables like the ones listed here is important to getting enough plant fibers.

Recommended vegetables

Asparagus	Carrots	Mushrooms	Romaine lettuce
Beets	Cauliflower	Mustard greens	Summer squash
Bok Choy	Collard greens	Okra*	Tomatoes
Broccoli	Eggplant*	Parsley	Zucchini squash
Brussel sprouts	Green beans	Pea pods	
Cabbage	Mesclun greens	Red peppers	

* These two vegetables have a gooey starch component that is especially good for lowering cholesterol. Slice up some eggplant, brush or spray on a bit of olive oil and grill it. Cholesterol-lowering therapy can taste so good!

Grilled Eggplant

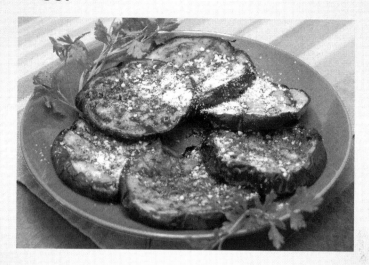

Directions

1. Wash a fresh eggplant, and slice into ½" thick slices, across the eggplant.

2. Brush or spray with olive oil.

3. Grill over medium hot coals ... turning every 3 – 4 minutes. Slices are cooked in about 10 minutes.

4. Season with balsamic vinegar, salt & pepper, tomato sauce or grated Parmesan cheese.

4. STARCHES: High fiber starches are nourishing and are good for both cholesterol and weight control.

Recommended starches

Black beans	Kidney beans	Pea beans	Pumpkin
Chickpeas	Lentils	Pinto beans	Sweet potatoes
Corn	Lima beans	Plantain	Winter squash
Hummus	Peas	Potatoes	

Some starches are especially high in fiber. Notice that black beans, kidney beans and lentils are all listed here as starches. People often think, "Oh, rice and beans; rice is the starch, and beans are the protein item." The amount of protein in a half-cup of beans is 7 grams, about equal to a one-ounce slice of turkey or cheese. Accompanying this 28 calories of protein is another 100 calories of starch. So while they offer a few more grams of protein per cup than most "starch" foods like corn and potatoes, still view beans, split peas, and lentils as starches. The extra protein and fiber content in beans makes them digest slowly, keeping blood sugar and insulin responses low as people assimilate them. They are the ultimate "low glycemic index" starch.

5. **GRAINS:** Whole grains have more fiber than white ones. Try:

Recommended grains

Barley	Corn tortillas	Oats/Cheerios	Soba noodles
Brown rice	Millet	Oat Bran	
Buckwheat	Quinoa	100% Rye bread	

Notice, *wheat* is not here in the recommended grains list. Wheat is a grain, and whole wheat is a possibility, but I am finding many people are more comfortable when they move away from eating wheat on a consistent basis. So yes, whole wheat bread has more fiber, but there is an issue of whether it promotes some inflammation, which would raise the risk of having cholesterol stick to arteries, and raise the incidence of having extra calories turn to abdominal fat more readily.[132] I also find in my clinical practice, having people eat less wheat, even whole wheat, reduces their acid reflux.

Two German fellows, Wolfganz Lutz, MS and Christian Allan, PhD., wrote a very interesting book called "*Life Without Bread.*"[133] It has many positive case reports of how people look and feel better after having stopped eating wheat and fewer grain foods in general. Their food plan is higher protein and lower carbohydrate as well, but particularly suggests that people be wary of grain. I am not advocating the avoidance of all grain, but I am urging people to use other carbohydrate sources like fruits and legumes more often. I am also suggesting that people eat barley, buckwheat, and quinoa more often, plus spelt and millet, when choosing grain calories.

A good advancement in eating style: become knowledgeable about preparing quinoa, and feel confident making some good-tasting dishes with it. Use it to make a salad, the way you would use pasta in a salad. Basically, have some cooked quinoa on hand, all chilled in the refrigerator. Add chopped vegetables and a dressing, and you're all set.

Quinoa Salad Recipe

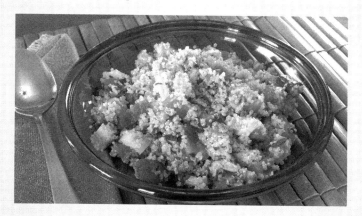

Quinoa boils up like rice; simply add twice the water for the amount of quinoa.

Ingredients

1 cup   Quinoa, uncooked

1   green or yellow pepper, diced

2   4" pickling cucumber (skin on), diced

1   small Vidalia onion or 6–8 scallions (tops & bottoms) diced

Dressing

1/3 cup   freshly-squeezed lemon juice

¼ cup   extra virgin olive oil

¾ cup   finely-chopped fresh cilantro or parsley

Directions

1.   Boil 1 cup quinoa in 2 scant cups water for 12-15 minutes.

—*continued on next page*

Quinoa Salad Recipe – continued

2. Now add vegetables, such as peppers and cucumbers, diced into ½ inch cubes.

3. Add onion or scallions and, if tomatoes are in season, and taste good, add one.

4. For dressing, whisk together 1/3 cup freshly-squeezed lemon juice and ¼ cup olive oil. Add in ¾ cup finely chopped fresh cilantro or parsley.

5. Pour dressing over the salad, and stir in. Serve warm, or let chill in refrigerator for a few hours.

Notes

- You can cook the quinoa ahead, and just chop vegetables and add to already chilled quinoa.

- One cooking note. Quinoa has a slight musty or ash flavor. I sauté an onion in a pot, add the quinoa and water, and add 1 bay leaf, then boil everything. The result is: no musty flavor.

6. NUTS & SEEDS: Essential fats found in nuts and seeds also help to reduce the risk of cardiovascular disease and to lower cholesterol numbers.[134] Cholesterol travels through the blood in protein/fat droplets called lipoproteins. These droplets hook up to lipoprotein receptors on the surface of cells lining arteries, the first step in moving cholesterol from arteries on into cells. Next, a lipoprotein "lipase" ushers the droplets through arterial walls, on into cells. The primary fuel to run the lipases/levers is a conditionally essential fat labeled gamma linolenic acid (GLA.)[135] This is a fat found mostly in seeds, (think pumpkin and sunflower first,) and in oil from plants like Evening Primrose and Borage. The body can convert a small amount of the fat in corn oil and vegetable oils—linoleic acid (LA) – into GLA, but direct sources in the diet are important too.

The tough fact is that people are too often told (erroneously) to avoid all fats to lower their cholesterol and their risk of heart disease. In the process they cut down on oils, and they certainly avoid seeds, which are known to be fatty.

So they end up having a deficiency of GLA, which is the oil that is the moisture barrier in the skin, as well as the fuel to support the lipase lever I just mentioned.

> Often people coming to me for cholesterol reduction advice have said, **"I don't understand it, the longer I am on my low fat and low cholesterol diet, the higher my cholesterol goes."**
>
> Then I've said, "And **tell me how dry your skin is.**"
>
> Eyes widened, they replied, "How did you know? My skin is incredibly dry. I have to use skin lotion all the time, and I hate it, especially in the winter when the skin on the ends of my fingers cracks and hurts."

In addition to a focus on the essential fat in seeds, many nuts still support lower cholesterol numbers. In most studies, almonds have some properties that lower cholesterol numbers.[136] Remember too, that nuts have many nutrients, like magnesium, that will help not only cholesterol numbers, but also help weight loss and blood sugar numbers in people with type 2 diabetes.[137] Walnuts also have added anti-inflammatory action on the cells lining arteries. [138]

Here is an example of a good clinical case, using fruits, probiotics, and essential fats to lower LDL cholesterol.

> Betty is a 61-year old woman who came to see me since she was hoping to avoid the Lipitor her doc wanted her to take. She was already eating a low cholesterol, low saturated fat diet. Her weight was normal. Her cholesterol was 301. Before you gasp, her HDL was 100. Her Cholesterol to HDL ratio is less than 3.5 to 1, so in one respect, her high cholesterol is offset by her tremendously high HDL. Framingham Heart Study data suggests the ratio is fine so her heart disease risk is low.[139] Her Triglycerides were normal, and her LDL was 178. She represents a dilemma. Some medical experts would say that the LDL must be lower, down to 159 no matter what. Remember, high cholesterol is a risk factor in premature heart disease, but she was over 60 and doing well. She took a small beta-blocker pill, not for hypertension, but to prevent her from an occasional too-rapid heart beat.

In discussing her diet, she agreed that she could eat 3 fruits a day, instead of the one to two she currently consumed. She said that her stools sank in the toilet. She did not have dry skin, though she consumed few seeds, and her main oil for cooking was olive, not a source of GLA.

I encouraged her to take one probiotic pill a day until her poop floated, (it took 2 weeks to achieve this result) and asked her to eat 3 fruits daily. Rather than consume sunflower and pumpkin seeds, which she didn't really care for, I suggested that she take 2 Oil of Evening Primrose pills a day, 1000 mg each, as a source of GLA. She would take these until she had her next cholesterol check. In 3 months she emailed me the results of her lipid check. It was nice news. Her total cholesterol was down a few points, but her LDL dropped 27 points, down to 163, and her HDL rose even higher, to 107! Her physician was happy with these numbers and said she could skip the prescription for Lipitor.

I still encouraged her to take 2 grams a day of fish oil, for the EPA/DHA to keep her arteries slippery, and to eat colorful foods, especially red grapes, so her cholesterol would not be oxidized and cause inflammation in her arteries, and to take an antioxidant multivitamin with 100 to 200 iu of "natural" vitamin E a day.

The good cholesterol news inspired her to spend a little more time on her bicycle too. Now her heart attack risk would drop even lower.

The bottom line … If you are over 60, and don't have heart disease, and your cholesterol number is up a little, rest assured that you can reduce your heart disease and heart attack risk with food and fitness activity. Again, your diet and exercise program is the most potent heart disease prevention therapy you can do, much more powerful than taking some medicine. If you are taking a statin drug, ask your physician if you can try a period without it, and see what numbers you can generate with your new knowledge of good fats, good fruit fibers, probiotics, and fitness activity.

Do the following and see how your numbers play out.

1. Exercise 30 minutes per day, 5 times a week.

2. You can eat the saturated fat of meat once or twice a week.

3. You can eat the saturated fat of cheese, in 1-ounce servings, once every 2 or 3 days.

4. Eat fruit three times a day.

5. Eat 2 to 3 cups of vegetables every day.

6. If not consuming fish 3 times a week, take one or two fish oil pills a day, to achieve 500 to 1000 mg intake of EPA/ DHA.

7. Take two Evening Primrose oil pills per day, 1000 to 1300 mg each.

8. Take a "probiotic" supplement often enough to get stools that generally float.

9. Take your antioxidant multivitamin daily, like the Active 50+ from Trader Joe's or take 1 to 2 pills of the Life Extension Foundation vitamin called Two Per Day Tablets or take the Simply One 50+ Men or 50+ Women multivitamin made by Super Nutrition.

Check your blood work in three months; see how good the results look.

Hypertension _____

Many people with hypertension end up on two or three medications to maintain control of their blood pressure. The side effects of pressure-lowering medicines include: fatigue, headaches, cough, swelling of hands or feet, muscle cramping, dizziness, lightheadedness and low potassium. Many people ask me about more natural solutions for treatment of hypertension.

Science Lesson

Fine muscles in the walls of arteries and veins contract and relax to maintain a certain amount of pressure in the vascular system. There are a number of hormone-like chemicals in blood vessels that regulate relaxation and contraction of those vessel wall muscles. As we age, the muscles and the cell walls of this vascular system may be a little less pliable. The assortment of chemicals that regulate fluid volume may operate with a little less precision.[140] Kidney function, which plays a role in regulating fluid volume in the vascular system, slows down.

Usual nutrition advice for lowering blood pressure is to reduce sodium level in the diet. The mineral sodium attracts water. Extra sodium in the blood and tissues brings in water and the added volume in blood vessels raises pressure in the plumbing network. It seems like there is sodium in everything: bread, pasta, milk, and cheese, not to mention cold cuts, soups and catsup. People often get frustrated trying to avoid it, and abandon their sodium reduction effort. Truly avoiding sodium seems difficult, and people just don't do real well with it.[141] Furthermore, the reward of being on a low sodium diet feels like a life of bland foods.

Interestingly, if the body can just do a better job pumping sodium back out of cells, then pressure drops back down. Researchers at The Brigham and Women's Hospital in Boston figured out that people consuming more of the minerals **magnesium, potassium, and calcium** excrete sodium better, and blood pressure does stay lower, even for people who don't eat strictly low sodium diets.[142] They have a website that details how to eat. What you'll notice there is that much of the dietary components are cave person food fundamentals. See details of the DASH diet at www.dashdiet.org.

An even more dynamic and focused intervention to lowering blood pressure naturally comes from the University of Vermont. In the book called *The K+ Factor* lead author, Richard Moore, PhD, points out that the ratio of Potassium (symbol K+) to Sodium (symbol Na+) in milk, nature's first food, is 3:1. His work has shown that if one eats a diet that has 3 parts K+ to 1 part Na+, it is quite hard to have an elevated blood pressure.[143]

A simple example: if you have a bowl of Cheerios, 160 mg sodium per cup, you have to offset that with 480 mg of potassium, which happens to be the amount in one banana.

Look in the tables below to see how the K⁺ Factor food plan would play out in a modern versus a Paleo era breakfast. See how you could concoct hypertension therapy for this meal. Notice, 2 slices of bread provide an average of 300 to 400 mg sodium, so you need 900 to 1200 mg K+ to offset the bread's Na+. A medium banana will provide the 500mg K+. A milk or yogurt is kind of a neutral: 375 mg K in a glass of milk, but 125 mg Na+. You still need to come up with 300 mg or so of potassium. An orange for a snack would do it.

Notice the mineral balance in a modern, grain-based breakfast, compared to the Paleolithic breakfast I encourage.

Modern Food Plan Breakfast

FOOD	SERVING	POTASSIUM	SODIUM	MAGNESIUM	CALCIUM
Whole wheat toast	2 slices	50	400	20	40
Smart Balance	2 tsp	3	60	0	0
Orange juice, fresh	4 oz	236	1	12	11
Coffee	10 oz	145	6	9	6
½ & ½	2 Tbsp	39	12	3	32
Sugar	2 tsp	0	0	0	0
Totals		473	479	44	89

The K+ Factor in modern breakfast is 0.987, a bit less than 1:1 ratio.

Paleolithic Breakfast

FOOD	VOLUME	POTASSIUM	SODIUM	MAGNESIUM	CALCIUM
Salmon	3 oz	369	49	28	38
Banana	1 large	487	1	37	7
Almonds	15 avg	127	0	48	48
Tea	10 oz	110	9	9	0
Milk	1 oz	43	13	3	36
Honey	2 tsp	7	1	0	1
Totals		1143	73	125	130

The K+ Factor here in an old world breakfast is 15.6 … almost a 16:1 ratio

If you at all wonder how well the K factor works, here is some proof. Six months into the initial publicity tour promoting *The K Factor*, its success was becoming apparent, corporate interests had forced MacMillan publishing to stop the book tour. http://www.minconf-forests.net/drug-books/richard-moore-md-phd-drugs-are-not-the-answer-for-high-blood-pressure!

Blood Sugar Levels Impact Blood Pressure Levels

Carbohydrate calorie loads are another nutrition connection to blood pressure to appreciate. When people eat fruits and starches, as those foods digest, blood sugar levels rise. Insulin tells cells around the body to open up and absorb sugar from the blood. However, insulin also has *build fat*, *retain sodium* and *make hungry* messages too. Think about a modern breakfast. By the time you add up the amount of carbohydrates from a typical breakfast: 2 slices of toast, plus a large banana and 4 ounces milk, you end up with 61 grams of carbohydrate: (30 toast, 25 banana, 6 milk). This is 244 carbohydrate calories. Insulin responds to rises in blood sugar and ends up telling the hormone aldosterone in the kidney to retain sodium.[144] In other words, blood pressure can go up when the size of carbohydrate servings are substantial or excessive. If breakfast were a caveman-era blend of protein-fruit-nuts, blood pressure would stay lower. If you make breakfast a whey protein and banana smoothie, plus a handful of almonds instead, there is less insulin expression. Having low sodium-low fat cottage cheese, a small banana, and 2 tablespoons of raw, unsalted sunflower seeds can also produce an impressive K:Na ratio (37:1) while keeping insulin response low.

See Diabetes section for more information on other insulin signals, like the "build fat" and "make hungry" messages that insulin generates.

The Heart as a Pump

Are you over 50 and looking for a little more energy? Think about providing your heart with a little more fuel. The heart pumps 5.6 liters of blood through the body in about 20 seconds! You may remember from some school science courses that fat and sugar are converted to the energy form called adenosine triphosphate (ATP) in the Krebs Cycle. ATP is the energy currency for muscles. This all happens in the mitochondria, small power plant units inside all the cells in the body, including cardiac cells. There is a vitamin-like substance called Coenzyme Q10 inside the mitochondria that completes the ATP production process. I call Co Q10 the velvet lining inside all the power plant units in the body, including cardiac cells.

As we age, Co Q10 levels can be less than optimal in our heart and other cells. We get Co Q10 in the protein foods we eat: fish, chicken, eggs and meats. This isn't quite enough to meet our needs. Usually, the liver converts the Co Q7, Co Q8 and Co Q9 found in fruits and vegetables to Co Q10 to complete the supply for our heart's needs. After age 50, the liver simply doesn't do this so well. Supplementation may be needed.[145] Also, statin drugs, commonly used to lower cholesterol, reduce Co Q10 production in the liver.[146] So age, plus taking certain medicines, compromise the ability of the liver to supply heart tissue with adequate Co Q10 for best energy production. If you are looking for a little more daily energy, you might want to discover what taking a Co Q10 supplement may do for you. See if you feel better taking it. You will not have zoom energy, like drinking coffee; this is just basic well-being energy, at no risk. If you are taking medicines to manage your blood pressure and you start taking Co Q10, be aware that you will likely need to lower your medicine doses in a few weeks.

Each day, blood travels 12,000 miles and the heart beats 10,000 times. Clearly, fuel levels for the muscle fibers in the heart matter. The quality of the heart's blood pumping contractions is measured as *ejection fractions*. Having lower Co Q10 levels in the heart mean less ejection oomph.[147] Interestingly, not long after age 20, liver production of Coenzyme Q10 starts waning a bit.[148]

Karl Folkers, a researcher at the University of Texas, was the man who first described the chemical structure of Coenzyme Q10, in the late 1950's.

He conducted a number of trials, using Coenzyme Q10 supplementation in many cardiac cases. The routine result was that ejection fractions improved. Another consistent effect was that people reduced the amount of blood pressure medication they were taking.[149] If you are taking several hypertension medicines and would like to explore how to reduce your need for them, look into taking 200 mg a day of Co Q10. Check blood pressure daily, and see how much it goes down. Again, you may need to reduce prescription drug doses. Adding 200 to 400 mg a day of magnesium could be beneficial as well.

Just so you know, Coenzyme Q10 has other benefits. It is a potent antioxidant, so it has a role in keeping blood vessels of people with diabetes, even those treated with a statin medicine, in better shape.[150] It is also fuel for a set of immune cells called Natural Killer cells.[151] These cells play a role in the body's fight against invading viruses and other germs. Its use, along with some other antioxidants has helped people with breast cancer have better remission rates when on a breast cancer chemotherapy treatment program.[152] Most people taking it find that they have a bit more energy in their day-to-day life. Finally, there is no risk to health in taking it. Coenzyme Q10 will not interfere with other prescription medicines, but you likely will need to reduce some blood pressure medication doses. Please check in with your doctor.

Mike is a guy who has had Type 1 diabetes for 46 years. Long term diabetes can cause kidney damage and Mike was no exception. He was already taking 2 types of insulin, plus Lipitor for his cholesterol, and thyroid replacement hormone. His blood pressure was high, even though he was taking 3 different medicines to lower it, plus doing acupuncture and tai chi. I suggested he try Coenzyme Q10, 100 mg a day. Within a few weeks his pressure dropped 20 points, settling into the low 120's.

Heart Failure
Common Nutrient Failures

As already mentioned, the heart is a muscle that weakens as we age. The muscle is simply not working so well. One consequence is reduced ability to pump fluids around the body, especially blood. Picture the image: blood is pulled to the feet by gravity, but cardiac contractions must push the blood up from the feet, back through the veins to the heart. If the pump is sluggish, fluid pools in the ankles and lower legs. The medical answer is to use a drug like Lasix, "a fluid pill" that keeps people a little drier with less fluid to leak into the extremities.

Anyone with the swollen ankles of heart failure knows it is downright annoying and painful. Swollen tissue hurts. Imagine the swelling of bee stings around both ankles all day and night. Anything that could be done to prevent this is worth knowing about. Coenzyme Q10 at 200mg a day is a good start to reducing ankle swelling in heart failure patients.

Here are some quotes from an abstract published in a congestive heart failure journal:[153] I can't emphasize enough how hugely dynamic smart nutrition intervention can help people in this condition.

Title: *Nutritional assessment in heart failure patients.*

Journal: Congest Heart Fail. 2011; 17(4):199-203

Authors: Lee JH, Jarreau T, Prasad A, Lavie C, O'Keefe J, Ventura H.

Source: John Ochsner Heart and Vascular Institute, Ochsner Clinical School, The University of Queensland School of Medicine, New Orleans, LA, USA.

Abstract: Heart failure (HF) is a growing epidemic worldwide with a particularly large presence in the United States. Nutritional assessment and supplementation is an area that can be studied to potentially improve the outcomes of these chronically ill patients.

.... **Coenzyme Q10**, a key component in the electron transport chain, is vital for energy production. **L-carnitine**, an amino acid derivative, is responsible for transport of fatty acids into the mitochondria along with modulating glucose metabolism. **Thiamine** and the **other B vitamins**, which serve as vital cofactors, can often be deficient in HF patients. **Omega-3 fatty acid** supplementation has been demonstrated to benefit HF patients potentially through anti-arrhythmic and anti-inflammatory mechanisms. **Vitamin D** supplementation can potentially benefit HF patients by way of modulating the renin-angiotensin system, smooth muscle proliferation, inflammation, and calcium homeostasis. ..... more studies are needed to solidify these recommendations.

When it comes to nutritional care in heart failure, most studies intervened with just 1 nutrient. When the heart cells are low in 4 to 5 items, clearly a single nutrient won't help much.

There have been a few small combo studies, but the results look good. The author Jeejeebhoy, in the abstract below, is a giant in the world of sophisticated nutritional studies.[154] Again, I want to quote some sections of the research abstract so you don't miss them.

Title: *Conditioned nutritional requirements: therapeutic relevance to heart failure.*

Journal: Herz. 2002; 27(2):174-8.

Authors: Sole MJ, Jeejeebhoy KN.

Source: University of Toronto, Toronto, Canada.

Abstract

BACKGROUND:

… Several specific metabolic deficiencies have been found in the failing myocardium: (1) a reduction in L-carnitine, coenzyme Q10, creatine, and thiamine--nutrient cofactors important for myocardial energy production; (2) a relative deficiency of taurine, an amino acid integral to intracellular calcium homeostasis; (3) increased myocardial oxidative stress and a reduction of antioxidant defenses.

METHOD AND RESULTS:

We have demonstrated deficiencies in carnitine, taurine and coenzyme Q10 in cardiomyopathic hamster hearts during the late stage of the cardiomyopathy. …. We also documented **carnitine, taurine and coenzyme Q10** in biopsies taken from **human failing hearts**, the levels correlating with ventricular function. A double-blind, randomized, placebo-controlled trial of a supplement containing these nutrients, given for 30 days, restored myocardial levels and resulted in a significant decrease in left ventricular end-diastolic volume.

CONCLUSION:

These experiments suggest that a comprehensive restoration of adequate myocyte nutrition may be important to any therapeutic strategy designed to benefit patients suffering from congestive heart failure. …

Compound Nutritional Support For Impaired Hearts

What people need to appreciate is that heart failure is not just about the heart. It is a systemic condition, characterized by much inflammation and inadequate repair materials. Repair materials in short supply can be items like low vitamin B2 and B6 levels.[155] Lower levels of sulfur compounds like cysteine are also an element of inadequate repair in the heart.[156] At the same time, the clean-up system is struggling. In a simple explanation, circulation is compromised, so toxins build up and so do stray electrons. There is more cytokine (chemical messengers that regulate clean-up) activity which generally leads to a feeling of fatigue. Cytokine messages also can contribute to insulin resistance. There can be a Catch-22 situation, as elevated blood sugars also trigger inflammation and vascular dysfunction.

Smart nutrition comes to the rescue. As you have already been reading, any time food and vitamins can reduce inflammation, people generally feel better and their bodies function better. Reversing heart failure is the finest example of how sophisticated nutritional support can make a wonderful difference in quality of life. Science is sometimes looking at glutathione peroxidase levels (a key antioxidant enzyme) in people with heart failure. This is a major antioxidant enzyme for the whole body. Its competence depends on adequate levels of protein and antioxidant nutrients like vitamin C, vitamin E, selenium and cysteine intake. This is a reminder that your Paleo-style diet and smart multivitamin supplement are fundamental.

You have already read about B-complex vitamins, Vitamin D and omega-3 fats in the previous pages. You are likely to be eating them in your food, and getting some extra amounts in your better-than-average multivitamin supplement. Taking Coenzyme Q10 is an important supplement introduced in this section.

So, heart failure is simply the heart not pumping enough. It can be due to age, corrosion or other damage. It can also result from not having enough fuel to pump as vigorously as it once did. Again, if you are feeling like your heart needs some more ooomph to manage fluids in your ankles more effectively give Coenzyme Q10 supplementation a try. See what kind of energy improvement you experience too. Take 100 mg, twice a day for 4 to 6 weeks. After that, 100 mg just once a day will likely be enough to maintain good energy.

Important, inform your physician that you want to take Co Q10 supplements for energy. There is no toxicity to Co Q10. The issue is that when it starts working for you, you may need to reduce the amount of heart regulation medicine you are taking. See the anecdote below.

> **With heart failure, a person's basic strength keeps dropping. Added nutritional support generally means people feel added energy, which improves quality of life.**

With poor circulation, cells lining the intestine are also at risk for not functioning properly. The gut's barrier function is compromised and debris (science words: endotoxin or lipopolysaccharide) from inside the intestines, circulates throughout the blood stream, and causes inflammation. As part of helping reduce all-over inflammation in the body of someone with congestive heart failure, (CHF), think of how the gut is doing. It merits nutritional attention.[157] See Gut Ecosystem in the next section for more info on this topic.

Here Is An Interesing Heart Failure Case

An 80-year-old man was sent to see me when he was told the elevations in blood sugar were nearing the diabetic level. He was already taking medicines for blood pressure, heart failure and atrial fibrillation, plus Lipitor for cholesterol. His heart was weak and his ankles often swelled with fluid. He was taking the fluid pill furosemide (Lasix) to reduce the pooled water in his lower legs. He hoped to avoid adding even more medicines for diabetes so he wanted to try managing his blood sugars with better diet.

I outlined a caveman style diet for him, which included a cottage cheese with banana and walnuts breakfast. Lunch remained a simple tuna or turkey sandwich, since that is what the local deli near his office could provide. Supper almost nightly became a baked potato or sweet potato, plus 1 to 2 cups of green vegetables. These provided potassium to push the sodium out of his system. I also urged him to eat salmon a few days a week, so the fish oils would keep the electrical part of his heart healthy.

I asked him to take a better antioxidant multivitamin that included stronger B complex, plus 100 mg magnesium, and 100 mcg selenium. I also started him on 100 mg Coenzyme Q10 twice a day for 3 weeks, then tapered to once a day for maintenance. Remember now, his age, and his being on a statin drug meant his Coenzyme Q10 levels were going to be at risk. His heart began pumping better, thanks to the Co Q10. After 3 weeks, he no longer needed the Lasix fluid pill. His doctor also lowered his blood pressure medicine dose too.

I have had this same experience with dozens of patients. Within 3 to 4 weeks of taking Coenzyme Q10, blood pressure is naturally lower, and BP medicines are reduced. It mimics the exact results of a Carl Folkers clinical trial that I want to quote here.[158]

Title: *Usefulness of coenzyme Q10 in clinical cardiology: a long-term study.*

Authors: Folkers K et al. Journal: Molecular Aspects of Medicine; 1994. 15 Supplement, pages 165-75.

"Before treatment with CoQ10, most patients were taking from one to five cardiac medications. During this study, overall medication requirements dropped considerably: 43% stopped between one and three drugs."

These are tremendous results! Taking less medication means fewer side effects. Plus, people feel an improvement in their basic energy level.

His blood sugars normalized. It was probably a combination of elements that helped the sugars improve. Better eating kept the blood sugar lower in general. A better vitamin helped insulin talk to muscle insulin receptors. Co Q10 made for better heart function; so better blood flow helped clear out metabolic waste in the body, which lowered cytokines that can cause insulin resistance.

It is a Catch-22 with heart failure. People feel weak, and exercise less, but more fitness activity would lead to better conditioning and improve well-being. I will say it again:

"Coenzyme Q10 is good for reversing fatigue in people with heart disease."

Nutrition can help break the cycle: low energy prevents the exercise that improves energy and conditioning. All kinds of athletes take the amino acid **L-glutamine**, to improve muscle repair after workouts, and improve performance during training. You already know it is a good idea to be taking **omega-3 EPA/DHA** for general health and brain function. A study at Columbia-Presbyterian Hospital in New York showed that taking these two supplements improved exercise capacity in people with CHF. Again, consult a professional for weaving these nutrition items into your current medical regimen.[159]

Conclusion: when feeling sluggish and frustrated because of heart failure, find a dietitian who can inform you of a careful intervention with a mineral-rich diet, plus a few key nutrients: Coenzyme Q10, antioxidant multivitamin, L-glutamine and L-carnitine. Discover how these supplements will improve your quality of life.

Food That Is Therapeutic Can Be Colorful And Tasty

Here is a cabbage and quinoa salad that lasts a few days in the refrigerator.

Quinoa Slaw with Thai Flavors
Recipe makes: approx. 8 cups

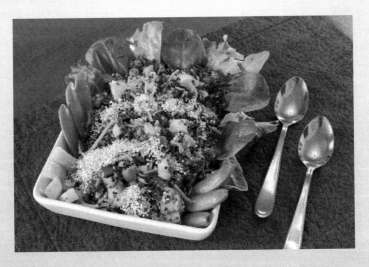

Ingredients

For the slaw:

1 cup	quinoa (black is fun if you can find it)
2 cups	water
2 cups	red cabbage, shredded
1 cup	snap peas, bias cut
1 cup	carrots, shredded

—Continued on next page

Quinoa Slaw with Thai flavors – continued

1 cup	scallions, bias cut
1 cup	mango, diced
1 cup	pineapple in small chunks
½ cup	clementine or orange pieces
½ cup	fresh cilantro, roughly chopped
¼ cup	sunflower seeds

Sesame seeds, toasted, to garnish

For the dressing:

½ cup	orange juice
¼ cup	rice wine vinegar
2 Tbsp	fresh ginger, minced
¼ cup	sesame oil
1 tsp	hot pepper sauce … optional

Instructions

1. One cooking note. Quinoa has a slight musty or ash flavor. I sauté an onion in a pot, add the quinoa and water, and add 1 bay leaf. Boil for 12 to15 minutes. The result is: no musty flavor.

2. In a bowl, stir together orange juice, rice wine vinegar, ginger and hot sauce. Slowly whisk in sesame oil to create an emulsion. Set aside to allow flavors in dressing to develop.

3. In a salad bowl combine quinoa, red cabbage, snap peas, carrots, scallions, mango, pineapple, orange/clementine and cilantro.

4. Fold in dressing and chill in fridge. When ready to serve, garnish with toasted sesame seeds.

Intestinal Health

Think about it: in a group of older people, hanging around chatting, the conversation frequently turns to gastrointestinal difficulties. Remember the Aunties in the play "Arsenic and Old Lace?" One complained of dyspepsia, and everyone knew what she meant.

The stomach and intestines are a complex metabolic system. The gastrointestinal system (GI system) is an approximately 40-foot-long tube running through the body. After people swallow food, it's on its way to the toilet, unless it digests down to molecular particles that are small enough to pass across the cell walls of the gut on into the blood stream. Think of the skin on your cheeks: the cheeks at either end of the body even! The skin rounds the corner and becomes the lining of the throat, gut, and colon. It's the skin either down the throat or up the butt. It now becomes very specialized in its function. It must allow selected food particles into the body across the intestinal wall. Then a little farther down the tube, it has to prevent some nasty crap from entering the body. These are quite a sophisticated set of cells. Clearly, you want that skin (cell layer) fiercely well nourished, so it can perform its job well.

A significant number of people experience intestinal system dysfunction. Irritable Bowel Syndrome (IBS) affects about 15% of the US population. The heartburn associated with acid reflux disease hits 60 million people once a month, and 25 million people are suffering daily according to The National Institute of Health. The problem of constant constipation affects 10% of the population, as reported by the National Health and Nutrition Examination Survey. Colitis, extra immune and nervous system activity, that results in the failure of intestine cell walls to adequately repair, is a common problem too.[160]

The incidence of GI dysfunction increases with age.[161] Sometimes it is unclear if the problems are an issue of aging physiology, or a side effect of other treatments. For example, many medicines have a constipating side effect.[162]

Science Lesson
The Gut Ecosystem

Picture the GI tract as a 40-foot long tube with its own ecology system. There are several hundred species of bacteria and microbes living there. The system has more nerve receptors for the neurotransmitter serotonin than does the brain. There are many immune cells produced in the Gut Associated Lymph Tissue (G.A.L.T.). The friendly bacteria in the gut, termed the *gut flora*, generate many of the nutrients that nourish cells lining the small and large intestines, and even the cells in other locations, like the lungs. The status of this ecosystem affects many body parts, not just gut comfort.

Diet plays a crucial role in establishing the breadth of the microbial array in the gut. Roughage, *i..e* the indigestible fiber in plants, is the groceries for the gut flora. A diet rich in fruit fibers, like pectin, plus the beta glucan fibers found in oats and legumes, (kidney beans, lentils and chickpeas), supports a bigger population of desirable microbes.[163] These beneficial microbes suppress the growth of noxious gut bugs, like yeasts and staph bacteria. The right or wrong set of gut flora also impacts tendency to gain weight and to develop diabetes.[164 165] You have already read about how good gut bacteria make small fat particles that help reduce cholesterol production in the liver. These small fat droplets are important repair fuel for cells lining the colon too. When people are experiencing "colitis," part of their problem can be lack of good gut flora, so there may be a deficiency of colonic cell repair material.[166] In general, people with a good gut flora population in their GI ecosystem will have stools that float in the toilet when they have a bowel movement. I tell people "fruit-fiber-floaters" when it comes to their gut health. If you are not eating your 3 fruit servings a day, then it is hard to consider you nourished in general. At the same time, I'd suspect your good gut flora are at risk of starving, and worry that your colon cells were not in their best state of repair. This means the ability of the colon to act as a tight barrier holding back bad news bugs from seeping into the body is at risk. I remind people, they are really just one flush away from the local sewer system. Yup, clearly gut flora quality matters.

There are supplements available that people can take to install a set of good gut bugs in their gut. The term "probiotic" refers to these beneficial microbe pills. Think of them as the opposite of antibiotics, hence: *pro*biotics.

Probiotics

Many items that people ingest can disrupt the gut ecosystem. The artificial sweetener sucralose seems to reduce good flora population.[167] Consuming too much alcohol is disruptive too.[168] Acid blocker drugs, like omeprazole, can shift flora pattern to higher population of Escherichia coli (E coli) and Candida albicans (yeast) species.[169] This is not good. Older people taking these acid reduction medicines experience higher rates of pneumonia, presumably from the change in gut flora patterns as well.[170]

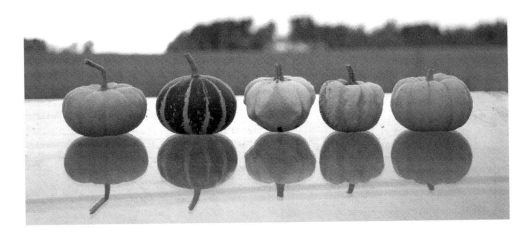

Having a comfortable bowel movement most days of the week is important.

Building A Better Bowel Movement

1. **Eating enough fruit fiber** is the first step toward assuring comfortable bowel movements. Fruit pulp nurtures a nice gut flora population. For this, be sure you eat fruit three times a day.

   - A banana a day is a good idea. No, they are not constipating or fattening. They do offer great fiber, which solves both constipation and diarrhea. A medium banana is 100 calories, not too fattening. Have a handful of nuts or seeds with any fruit to slow its digestion, if blood sugar is a concern.

   - An apple (or pear) a day does keep the doctor away.[171] Applesauce and canned pears work too.

   - A serving of berries is a good idea too, as both GI system and brain food.

2. If you suffer from constipation or diarrhea problems, and your doctor has ruled out major infection as a cause, consider taking a probiotic. A very good product to start with is *Culturelle* (see www.culturelle.com). It has been used in over 125 clinical trials, ranging from resolving diarrhea in children in Bangladesh to treating a mom to heal her nursing baby's eczema. Take it for 4 weeks. After that you should consider taking a probiotic that is a blend of Lactobacilli and Bifidobacter species.[172] A capsule that delivers

5 billion "colony forming units" is a good place to start. I have seen good clinical results with a product called *JarroDophilus EPS*.[173] It is a reasonably priced product that works for people. Take a probiotic for a week or two. Once stools float, you can take it less often, or stop it altogether, until sinkers happen, or until some gut symptoms return.

3. **The amino acid L-glutamine**, sold in powder form, is repair material for the cells lining the intestines. If you need to optimize the repair function in your GI system, try taking ½ teaspoon of L-glutamine once or twice a day. You can progress to a full teaspoon, taken once or twice a day. See how it makes you feel. Just put the ½ teaspoon, 2.5 grams dose, L-glutamine powder on your tongue and wash it down with a gulp of water. It is tasteless. It is often energizing. You may also feel a bigger zoom from your coffee and other caffeinated beverages when taking L-glutamine.

   • Only one precaution: pregnant women should not take L-glutamine. It has noot been studied in this group.

   • Read more about L-glutamine in the next section: a GERD remedy.

   • If you want more details of glutamine and cell repair, read an excellent book by Judy Shabert, RD, MPH, MD called Glutamine, The Ultimate *Nutrient*, published by Avery.[174]

Help With Acid Indigestion, Acid Reflux, and GERD

Acid reflux can occur in people of any age. Usual treatment is drugs that limit acid release in the stomach. The common ones are proton pump inhibitors and H2 agonists, but these medicines can adversely impact gut flora. Recent medical journal articles are mentioning that kidney damage from proton pump inhibitors is more common now that so many people are taking these drugs and for longer periods.[175]

It would be nice to see if the acid regulation system could be re-set to work properly. The following plan has helped patients, young and old. Give it a try. It will cost you about $35 for this two-week experiment.

Reflux is fluid flowing in reverse, from the stomach up into the lower part of the esophagus. When stomach acid washes up there with the flow, it is called "acid reflux".

Why this happens is not well understood. In part, the valve at the top of the stomach does not close enough, and acidic fluids leak upward. So far, the medical management goal is to stop the acid part of the backwash, so that no damage from the acid occurs. Acid corroding the cells of the lower esophagus for too long can cause scarring and cancer, so people take acid blocker drugs, like omeprazole (Prilosec). Just an FYI, long term use of those drugs can sometimes lower vitamin B12 levels in the body[176], and increases risk of osteoporosis,[177] and cause kidney damage. In aging acid production naturally declines, so excess acid production is puzzling. Meanwhile, it seems that use of acid-lowering drugs can provoke more acid production.[178] Acid blockers mess up the balance of friendly and not so friendly flora in the gut, increasing the incidence of pneumonias in older people. If using these medicines long term, try to keep the dose as low as possible.

The system that regulates stomach acid production is located in the cells lining the stomach. Acid release is one way the body disinfects food entering the GI system. In the olden days, foraging in the forest, food wasn't as clean as what we eat now; it seems that the body developed stomach acid as a way to disinfect what we ate. When stomach acid has done its job, acid production is supposed to stop. So why is there excess acid? Some researchers feel that if acid production isn't quite high enough, the gut keeps on churning out more acid. An analogy: the leaky toilet tank that keeps running because it never hits the high water mark, and never shuts itself off. A popular home remedy that many people find useful for treating acid reflux is to consume a teaspoon of apple cider vinegar at the end of a meal, to theoretically contribute a little more acid. I have no clinical experience with this, but so many people I've met have reported that it worked for them I feel like it is an idea worth passing on. There is a big volume of internet testimonials that says it's helpful too. If you try the vinegar, don't mix it with bicarbonate agents like Mylanta or TUMS. The common dose of apple cider vinegar is 1 teaspoon in 8 ounces of water. You want apple cider vinegar, like Bragg's brand, with the "mother" (a cloudy filament) floating in the bottom of the jar. My sense about this therapy is that it is fixing bacterial overgrowth in the intestines, not that it is adding useful stomach acid.

Another excess acid idea: wheat proteins may be the culprits. The version of wheat currently grown is hybridized Triticum. In earlier times, this wheat protein was diploid – a 2 chromosome protein. The current versions being grown are hexaploid and octoploid, 6 and 8 chromosomes, for better crop yield, resistance to disease, and special cooking properties. This modern wheat can be very irritating to intestine cells. Many people are finding out that avoiding wheat keeps their gut systems happier.[179] Avoiding "wheat" here means both white and whole wheat. It means the grain called wheat, as opposed to other grains like corn, barley, rye, and millet.

As part of the structural changes that gut cells make in response to the chronic stress of wheat irritation, they somehow generate acid-secreting signals. One of the possible interventions is to stop eating wheat for a while so this acid release message system fades away. Avoiding wheat is not the same as avoiding all gluten, a protein found in wheat, rye, spelt, and barley. However, it means no wheat, as in no regular muffins, pasta, bagels, crackers, cakes and cookies though. After a few weeks, it may be ok to eat some wheat again, but not on a daily basis.

Another theory that is gaining strength about the cause of reflux blames the excess fermentation in the intestines. So we are back to dyspepsia, burping, and too much intra-abdominal pressure.[180][181]

The nutrition concept here, then, is to get the whole gut ecology system in its best shape, so that the pancreas and the repair cells lining the gut are working optimally.

The next two pages present my two-week Reflux Remedy plan. After the two week trial, you might consider trying to reduce your dose of acid reflux management pills.

If you are one of the people who does not respond well enough to the Reflux Remedy plan, don't worry. You can try a more therapeutic food plan. It is a food scheme mapped out in a book called *Dropping Acid*.[182] It is a rigorous plan of avoiding acidic foods for several months. Even apples are acidic in this plan. It is not easy, but is quite effective.

Acid Reflux Remedy
Food and Nutrition Supplements for Gut Ecology

A Reflux Remedy Plan

Step 1: Eat a lot of water-soluble fibers. Start with eating 3 to 4 servings of fruit per day. Ideally among those fruit encounters, you eat one banana, and either one apple or one pear each day. These fruits have the most pectin. They can be fresh, frozen, canned or dried: ingesting more pulp fiber is the goal.

- Besides fruit, try for another dose of therapeutic fiber almost every day. Try having a tablespoon of ground flax, adding it to applesauce or yogurt. It tastes nutty. The fiber in flax nurtures gut flora.

- Another useful fiber to try eating every few days is oat bran. It cooks up like cream of wheat. It's a decent cereal. It is great as a mid-morning snack. Use Cheerios or oatmeal on other days. Bake yourself some oat bran muffins as a mid-morning snack. Quaker has a wonderful oat bran recipe at their website: http://www.quakeroats.com/cooking-and-recipe/oat-bran-muffins.aspx. Here is the recipe. View these muffins as medical nutrition therapy in a fun snack form.

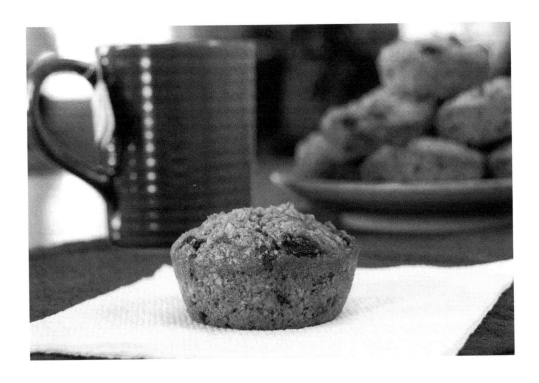

Quaker® Oat Bran Muffins

Ingredients

2 cups	Quaker® Oat Bran hot cereal, uncooked
¼ cup	Brown sugar, firmly packed
2 tsp	Baking powder
½ tsp	Salt
1 cup	Fat free milk or 2% reduced fat milk
2	Egg whites, slightly beaten
¼ cup	Honey or molasses
2 Tbsp	Coconut oil
1 cup	Raisins
¼ cup	Chopped walnuts

Serving Tips

Stir into batter ½ cup fresh or frozen blueberries or ½ cup mashed ripe banana

Preparation

1. Heat oven to 425° F.
2. Line 12 medium muffin cups with paper baking cups, or spray bottoms only with no-stick cooking spray.
3. Combine dry ingredients; mix well.
4. Add combined milk, egg whites, honey and oil; mix just until dry ingredients are moistened.
5. Add walnuts and raisins, mix until just combined.
6. Fill prepared muffin cups ¾ full.
7. Bake 15 to 17 minutes or until golden brown.

Step 2: Take some beneficial gut bacteria pills, sometimes called "probiotics". A brand I recommend is JarroDophilus EPS pills (25 bil CFU model). Take 1 per day.

Step 3: Take some L-glutamine each day. Glutamine is gut cell repair fuel. It is also immune cell fuel. It helps buff up the intestinal ecosystem in a variety of ways.

- 1 Tablespoon of L-glutamine powder provides 14 grams. You want to take 14 grams, twice a day, for about 2 weeks. Just dissolve the glutamine in an ounce of cool water or juice and drink it down. Don't mix it in anything hot. Take it 5 minutes before breakfast and dinner.

- If you are a coffee drinker or consuming a lot of caffeine in sodas, you may notice that you will get more of a caffeine buzz when taking glutamine. As I have mentioned before, pregnant women should not take glutamine, as it is un-studied in this population.

- If you have Crohn's disease or rheumatoid arthritis or other immune-related diseases, glutamine is actually beneficial. In autoimmune cases though, start the L-glutamine gradually, say ½ teaspoon a day for 3 days, and then increase by 1 teaspoon every 3 days. Note, 3 teaspoons equals 1 Tablespoon. The whole gut cell repair process will take longer for you then. Once up to the 1 Tablespoon of glutamine taken twice a day, then start taking the probiotic Culturelle for 4 weeks. Then progress to a probiotic that is a blend of species for a few weeks.

Again, after two weeks of extra good nutrition for gut cells, you can try reducing your reflux management pills. Don't just quit taking them; you have to stop gradually. If you feel better, but are not totally without symptoms, you might need a longer therapeutic program. Sometimes people have a more complex case of gut microbial imbalance (dysbiosis) that takes longer to reverse.

Reputable Supplement Source

Go to www.vitaminshoppe.com to buy the probiotic JarroDophilus EPS pills. They also have good prices on L-glutamine. You'll need a 400-gram container of glutamine for the 2 to 3 week therapeutic trial. The Jarrow company makes a good quality L-glutamine powder, so does Caged Muscle.

A Paleolithic Food Plan without wheat might look like this. (Adjust portion sizes to meet your caloric and appetite needs. This one provides approximately 1900 calories.)

Paleolithic Food Plan

MEAL	FOOD	CALORIES
BREAKFAST		
protein:	2 oz turkey, 3 Tbsp protein powder or 1/2 cup cottage cheese	100
fruit:	a small banana, 3/4 cup fresh or canned fruit	80
nuts:	1 Tbsp peanut butter or a handful of nuts or seeds	100
dairy:	6 oz Greek yogurt or 8 oz nut milk	80
bev:	black coffee, regular or green tea (optional)	
SNACK		
starch:	1 cup oatmeal or 1½ cups Cheerios	150
or fruit:	a small box of raisins or 1 cup applesauce	100
bev:	4 oz glass of almond milk	40
LUNCH		
protein:	3 oz salmon, sardines, turkey or chicken	150
starch:	1/2 cup kidney beans or lentils or 1 cup peas or potatos	150
veggies:	2 large carrots, or a tomato and a green pepper	60
SNACK		
dairy:	8 oz nut milk, or 1/2 cup Greek yogurt	80
SNACK		
nuts:	1 handful (2 Tbsp) walnuts, almonds, cashews	100
fruit:	a large peach, 3/4 cup pineapple chunks, or 1 medium apple	75
DINNER		
protein:	4 oz broiled fish, poultry, or lean meat	200
starch:	1 cup green peas, corn, limas, baked potato	150
veggies:	1 to 2 cups broccoli, cauliflower, spinach, carrots, etc.	80
oil:	1 Tbsp nuts, 1 tsp butter or 1 tsp olive oil	45
SNACK		
fruit:	a big orange or apple, or 2 plums or 2 kiwi fruits	100
dairy:	8 oz 1% fat milk or ½ cup Greek yogurt	100

Total calories: **1940**

The maintenance plan to keep acid regulation going well is different for each person. Some people take just 1 probiotic pill, once a week and 1 teaspoon of L-glutamine every 3 to 4 days. Others need the supplements a bit more often. They usually have a wheat food treat, like a slice of pizza, a muffin or some pasta just once every 3 or 4 days.

Muffin in a Mug Recipe

for a mid-morning,
non-wheat snack ...

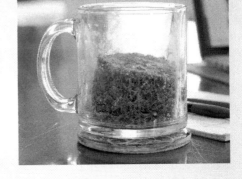

Ingredients

2 Tbsp ground flax seeds

2 Tbsp applesauce

½ tsp baking powder

1 tsp brown sugar

1 egg

Preparation

1. Mix 2 Tbsp Ground Flax seed with 2 Tbsp applesauce and ½ tsp baking powder, 1 tsp brown sugar, and 1 egg.

2. Season with cinnamon, nutmeg, ginger or apple pie spice blend.

3. Microwave on High, in a mug, for 75 seconds.

4. Let cool 2 to 3 minutes.

Perfect for a mid-morning fiber dose.

Diet For Diverticulosis

As people age, their gut walls are not as strong as they once were. People sometimes develop diverticuli, which are bulges or small pockets in the gut wall. The condition of having some of these bulges is called diverticulosis. For many years, a lack of fiber in the diet was considered to be the primary cause of diverticulosis, as it seemed that people eating more primitive (high fiber) diets did not develop the condition. A lack of insoluble fibers from grains and vegetables may contribute to development of divertulosis to some degree. Sometimes the bulges become infected, a condition called diverticulitis. A lack of water-soluble fibers from fruits seems to be part of the cause of the flare up.[183] However, more analysis shows that subtle inflammatory events, and even gut flora patterns are the more likely contributors.[184]

The best diet for diverticulosis is a high fiber one. Your primary challenge is to prevent constipation. Eat plenty of both **water-insoluble** and **water-soluble** fibers. Keep your intestinal ecosystem hydrated as well. You may know that caffeine and alcohol dry out your system, so after drinking dehydrating beverages you need to drink extra water and seltzers to restore your fluid level. Bowel movements should be routine and comfortable. The stools you pass should be spongy logs that generally float.

As an insurance policy to avoid constipation, people usually keep a bulking agent like Citrucel or Benefiber around. In the evening, take a moment to think about the food that you have eaten for the day. If you didn't eat the amount of fiber you usually do, take a dose of fiber supplement.

The goal of this food plan is also to get your gut ecosystem in good shape. Again, this means you nurture the growth of a good population of friendly, beneficial bacteria in your intestines. The good bacteria manufacture small fats that float your stools. They also produce antibiotics that support beneficial immune activity in the GI system. Remember, fruit fibers support good gut bacteria.

The Mediterranean Diet generally covers the food requirements. Consume generous portions of fruit at least 3 times a day, and add other high fiber foods like beans.

Some people with diverticulosis find there are certain foods they don't tolerate which cause pain and cramping. The skin on walnuts and peanuts, and on some fruits like grapes and apples may be bothersome. For other people, these foods are all fine, but cabbage and iceberg lettuce are intolerable. Specific food difficulties are generally unique to each person with diverticulosis.

One controversy in the diverticulosis diet is whether to avoid seeds. Raspberries, strawberries, tomatoes, cucumbers and popcorn have small seeds or other indigestible elements. Many people avoid these, believing the seeds will fall into the diverticuli and rot and cause infection: diverticulitis. This is a myth with no data to support it, and institutions such as the Mayo Clinic[185] and the Academy of Nutrition and Dietetics (formerly the American Dietetic Association) are now promoting high fiber diets.[186] Too many people are on restrictive diets that actually put them at higher risk for diverticulitis flares. Their restrictions keep people away from foods that are especially nourishing for the immune system.

If you are grocery shopping for you and your significant other, are you putting 42 fruit servings in your grocery cart this week? If not, bags of frozen berries and items like dried apricots and pineapple could help here.

Food shopping hint: if you are going to eat fruit 3 times a day to keep yourself nourished, you need twenty-one fruit servings for the week.

The bottom line is that the intestines cover an area the size of a tennis court and have serious nutritional needs. The cells lining the intestine wear out and are replaced every 4 to 5 days. If they are not repairing well, it is a major strain on the body. The GI system wants protein and a lot of good fibers to function well. You want to be familiar with how the use of probiotic and of L-glutamine supplements can help keep it in good condition. When this system is struggling, the whole body will also be struggling. The immune system will be challenged and asked to do more work. Muscles and skin will be neglected, as the GI system commands resources that would otherwise go for repair out around the body. Remember that you need 21 servings of fruit a week per person.

Crohn's and Colitis

For anyone dealing with Crohn's disease and ulcerative colitis, the gut nutrition information here is vital. The fruit, fiber, probiotic and L-glutamine information is especially important. Too many dietitians are focused on the concept "If you eat a good diet, you'll be fine". They have not learned enough about useful supplements. Physicians are trained to prescribe drugs. Prescriptions treat symptoms; they seldom support repair processes. The latest round of medicines for colitis are immune system suppressive. There is a higher risk of getting lymphoma when taking them!

I have a gastroenterology lecture called, "*Doctors Don't Know Shit*," meaning that doctors don't know the fine points of poop. Don't you get caught in the knowledge gap. Find a nutrition counselor who practices functional medicine, i.e., looks at the physiologic processes that will support gut repair. It will make a big difference. For chronic flare ups, include some Eastern medical treatment in your care routine. Give serious consideration to some acupuncture or Chigung or Tong Ren. You'll end up in much better shape.

Bone Health

Osteoporosis and Risk of Fractures

Osteoporosis is high on the list of American women's health concerns as they age. Bone scans are a routine part of preventative medical care for post-menopausal women. The Surgeon General's statistics indicate that 12 million people in America have osteoporosis and 40 million have low bone density to some degree.[187] The statistic that perhaps 20 percent of the people who suffer hip fractures are dead in the following 12 months is worrisome, as well.

As you know from your own life experiences there is a vast range in health status among people 60, 70, or 80 years old. Some people age 80 are out walking daily, while some 60-year olds are significantly impeded with arthritis, excess weight, and diabetes and heart conditions. A person's vigor or strength means more to their health prospects than any osteoporosis diagnosis. Robustness versus frailty is key when assessing risk for bone/hip fractures.[188]

Upon the first evaluation of your bone health with a bone scan, you might hear that your bones are thinner than the average 18-year old. Don't panic; the situation is not as dire as television and magazine ads would lead you to believe. Again, I defer to *Overdosed America*, where Dr. Abramson questions why we are compared to the body parts of an 18 year-old? As for how much to worry about osteoporosis, he reveals some interesting statistics in the Fosamax Study that led to the drug being approved by the FDA. Eight thousand (8,000) women enrolled to get either an active drug or a placebo. The women were 55 years of age and older. In the course of 4.2 years of study, **95.5%** of 4, 000 women taking a placebo remained fracture-free. On Fosamax, the number rose to only **95.8%** of 4,000 women being fracture-free.[189] Do you notice? The incidence of fractures is low to begin with, and the actual benefit accrues to just three-tenths of one percent (0.3 %) who take the drug for 4 years. Would you take a drug where you knew that just 1 person in 81 benefits in the course of 4.2 years? Would you ask about the side effects, like death of the jaw bone (osteonecrosis of the jaw) – which causes your teeth to loosen and wobble? Recent analyses point out Fosamax also increases some atypical leg fractures and advises just 3 to 5 years therapy at most.[190]

What I am most concerned about is that the focus on the low utility drug distracts people from alternate actions that can be far more useful in fracture prevention. There are a number of nutritional and fitness regimens associated with better bone health.

The true health concept is worry less about bone strength, and focus on preventing falls that result in fractures.

Key Elements For Preventing Fractured Bones[191]

- **Toned muscles:** People whose muscles have lost size and strength are more prone to falls. Eating enough protein is key to maintaining muscle volume. Doing resistance exercises, which means lifting weights or using exercise machines, maintains or even builds strength. A good test of functional muscle: can you stand from a chair without using your arms to get up?

- **Having a routine walking program** reduces risk of fractures. The longer the walks, the lower the risk. The opposite is true. Being too sedentary is a problem. People who are on their feet less than 4 hours a day are at more risk.

- **Tuned up proprioceptors:** Little sensors in the joints tell you what your arms and legs are doing: feeling muscle length and tone, and what angle your joints are at. You don't watch your legs and feet as you walk. You look forward and inherently know how far out you have placed your feet as you take steps. Your proprioceptors are letting your brain know what's going on in your limbs. You could eat with your eyes closed, and get the fork to your mouth thanks to the same sensors. Proprioceptors can lose their sensitivity from lack of movement. It's like a muscle where you use it or lose it. People who are very busy in their regular life, get caught up in chores and duties, where they miss their "daily walk" or exercise activity for 4 to 5 days. Even this is enough for people to experience a reduction in leg coordination. Routine fitness activity keeps proprioceptors tuned up. Lack of activity leads to poor function and less stability walking. Nursing home programs that have people doing even just 10 minutes a day of muscle activity, like calisthenics, walking, stepping, or stretching, see a major reduction in falls and fractures.

- **Being well-nourished** matters to bone strength. Get blood tests to be sure your Vitamin D levels are $\geq$ 50 nmol/L ($\geq$20 ng/ml). The DASH diet for blood pressure management, which emphasizes eating enough foods with calcium, magnesium and potassium, while limiting sodium, keeps bones stronger, too.[192]

- **Having better vision** helps prevent falls. Wearing glasses to maintain depth perception is important. Having cataracts, glaucoma and diabetic retinopathy increases risk for falls and fractures.

- **Having a mother who had a hip fracture** increases a woman's risk of fracture. This is the case regardless of bone density status. Clearly it is too late to change your family of origin but hopefully this information can inspire or motivate you to maintain fitness and nutrition habits that reduce other risk factors.

Osteoporosis and fracture rates are the highest in countries with the most milk and calcium intake. Daily calcium intake in the United States generally hovers around the 1000 mg mark, depending on what age and gender group you examine.[193] For example: in Beijing, women consume little milk and dairy and average about 587 mg calcium intake per day.[194] Chinese women have some of the lowest age-related fracture rates in the world.[195] With urbanization, the rates are doubling, and then some, for both men and women.[196] This would suggest something about doing less physical activity influences fracture rates. Interestingly, in another study of Chinese women better bone density was correlated to higher fish and fruit consumption.[197] One might speculate that the fish are helping vitamin D levels, and the fruit is nourishing the GI system, so there may be less inflammation in the body.[198] In Japan osteoporosis rates are about 8% of the population, similar to the US numbers. However, fracture rates are less than half what they are in the US.[199] Their calcium intake averages 400 to 500 mg a day, mostly coming from small fish with bones, soy products and vegetables. This data raises the question of whether milk and dairy are the best foods for assuring a calcium intake that would really help increase bone strength and reduce fracture risk? There's some study data on calcium and vitamin D, from dairy products, preventing fractures in the elderly,[200] but the true fracture prevention picture is far more complex.

Harvard Medical School and the Harvard School of Public Health offer their own version of the US government's "My Plate" for teaching healthy eating,[201] and it does not contain the small round glass of milk symbol that is part of the USDA "My Plate" nutrition advice program.[202] This leaves the impression that low intakes of vitamin D and trace minerals like magnesium are under-appreciated aspects of the thinning bones problem. The inflammation factor does not get enough attention either. Of course the practical food advice to cover all of these pitfalls is here in this book.

Knowing the exact amount of vitamin D, calcium, and other nutrients to eat to prevent or reverse osteoporosis is difficult. The Dietary Reference Intake (DRI) for vitamin D for seniors age 51 to 70 years is 600 iu/day, and for the elderly over 70 is 800 iu/day.[203] The recommended amounts for calcium are 1,000 mg for men under age 70, 1200 mg for women under 70, and 1200 mg calcium for everyone over 70.[204] These calcium numbers are now under some suspicion as being too high. There is some concern emerging about taking too much calcium in pill form. One Australian study detected more heart attacks in women taking calcium at 500mg per day.[205][206] Of course, one study should not change all clinical suggestions. Researchers tracking 23,980 Heidelberg area residents for about 11 years, as part of a diet and cancer study, suggest proceeding cautiously with supplements because of cardiac risks, versus regular dietary intake of calcium.[207]

If your bones are thin, and sometimes hurt, and you want to truly re-calcify them, look into the concepts outlined by the Algaecal company: www algaecal com. The bone remodeling (re-calcifying) data for their supplement trials is impressive. In a way, calcium from algae mimics the calcium from leaves that we got in the olden days. The Algaecal people generated good bone remodeling with 540 – 720 mg per day of supplemental algae-origin calcium, while depending on diet to supply about 700. The Algaecal company bone-rebuilding product includes a trace mineral supplement that provides boron, magnesium, and strontium, plus vitamin K2 and vitamin D. There are now other commercial products that mimic the Algaecal blend, available at your local vitamin shops. Thinner, porous bones can often hurt and this plant-based calcium-vitamin mineral cocktail looks like the best way to re-mineralize them.

However, remember that for preventing fractures there is an important role for bone strength and nutrition, but you must do more activity. In looking at 77,000 women enrolled in the Nurses Health Study, yes more calcium, vitamin D, and other minerals made stronger bones, but this was not enough for reducing fracture rates. [208][209] Bone mineral level is not a sole risk factor in fractures. Falling is the problem. That's about muscles and strength and co-ordination (and removing scatter rugs and other obstacles from floors).

A statement about fracture prevention from the Europeans … [210]

The European Society for Clinical and Economic Aspects of Osteoporosis and Osteoarthritis (ESCEO) recommends optimal dietary protein intake of 1.0 to 1.2 grams/kilogram bodyweight/

day with at least 20 to 25 grams of high-quality protein at each main meal, with adequate vitamin D intake at 800IU/d to maintain serum 25-hydroxyvitamin D levels >50 nmol/L as well as calcium intake of 1000 mg/d, alongside regular physical activity/exercise 3 to 5 times/week combined with protein intake in close proximity to exercise, in postmenopausal women for prevention of age-related deterioration of musculoskeletal health.

Bouncing Back from a Fracture

If someone you know experiences a fracture, jump into nutrition support mode. Supplements can play a dynamic role in reducing complications and speeding recovery after bone repair surgery. An 8-ounces drink with 254 calories and 20 grams of protein (supplemental drinks like Boost Plus or Ensure Plus) consumed once a day shortened convalescence from 40 to 24 days in one study. Complications to recovery, even 6 months later, were just 40% in the nutritionally supplemented people versus 74% in the others.[211]

Here is an interesting bit of research information. After a fracture, don't presume older age is an automatic detriment to recovery. In a Montreal study of 241 people, average age 75.4 years old, death rates after a hip fracture were higher in the people less than 70 years old, and lowest for people older than 80.[212] This brings us back to individual constitutional elements that determine health. Younger people having a fracture may already have been frail from some unknown reason.

Arthritis
Think Nutrition for less "Itis" and for More Joint Repair

Arthritis is complex. Interestingly, there is some evidence that lower birth weight, and lower weight at age 1 put people at higher risk for getting osteoarthritis.[213] While Traditional Chinese Medicine has viewed arthritis as involving Chi stagnation, with deficiency in liver (Gan) and kidney (Shen). It has also said there is an immune cell component. In fact, recent research points to varying levels of activated (immune system) CD4 T cells and Th17 cells in both osteoarthritis and rheumatoid arthritis.[214] Of course immune systems are sensitive to nutrition. Knowing that vitamin D has immune system functions, you may not be surprised to learn that people with low vitamin D levels have more arthritis pain and fatigue.[215]

Another view of arthritis is that repair activity in the cells of joints is not keeping pace with the wear-and-tear they are experiencing. Now one solution is to reduce wear and tear, and provide more repair nutrients. Another is to consider whether the body is too busy with rehab activities in other places, so that it cannot direct enough resources to the joint cells. Add to this scenario the concept that food is either helping or impeding the many repair systems throughout the body.

In treating both rheumatoid and osteoarthritis, people need first to take care of their **gut ecosystem**. If this is not in its best state of repair, then stuff "leaks" though the gut wall causing the body to be busy coping with that, leaving fewer resources for cleaning up joint spaces. Revisit the pages about fruit, fibers and probiotics to keep the gut ecosystem in good shape. The **eating fruit** part of the caveperson era diet outlined here is very much like the Mediterranean Diet, which is associated with lower rheumatoid arthritis (RA) symptoms.[216] Taking a probiotic supplement that contains 2 billion colony-forming units each of Lactobacillus casei, Lactobacillus acidophilus, and Bifidobacterium bifidum significantly reduced rheumatoid arthritis symptoms, and many inflammatory cytokines like Tumor Necrosis Factor *alpha*.[217]

In aging, repair processes are just slower than they were 20 or 30 years earlier in life. This can lead to body parts developing an "itis" where there is likely some extra inflammation and pain. To help reduce this "itis," think about the therapeutic use of **essential fats**. These are food elements that you would have been eating a bit more of, if you were living in a time before grains, chickens and cows were added to our routine diet. There are several levels of omega-3 EPA/DHA oil you can try.

- **Fish oil 3 grams a day** providing 1500 mg total EPA/DHA[218]

- **Fish oil, 2 grams a day** providing 1,000 mg total EPA/DHA and krill oil, 500 mg providing approx. 150 mg EPA/DHA[219]

- If not totally satisfied with the fish oil results add **Primrose oil, 2,000 mg** providing 200 mg GLA[220]

I also recommend an **antioxidant multivitamin**, and **L-glutamine at 5 grams** per day. The vitamin keeps the Omega fats chemically stable. The glutamine is important for assuring good osteoblast function.[221] Osteoblasts are the cells that renew bone matrix, depositing calcium in the mineral mix. Glutamine also helps gut cells maintain their barrier function.

Another compound that has dynamic effects on the "itis" regions of arthritis, and documented pain reduction action is **curcumin**.[222] This is the active compound in turmeric. Because this supplement is more herbal than nutritional when used in its effective doses I don't feel qualified to give advice about it. I also don't know it well enough to report precautions. I do know it is in the ginger family, so avoid it if you are allergic. I have seen the 900 mg per day dose be helpful for many people. Also, the combination of curcumin and resveratrol (grape extract) is also showing promise in arthritis management.[223]

Often some subtle food intolerances or sensitivities (not quite as dynamic as out-and-out food allergies) can play a role in arthritis symptoms. For people experiencing pain, despite taking all the previously mentioned supplements, I suggest avoiding various foods for a week or two at a time as an experiment.

To start, try 2 weeks of **eating no products made with wheat**. This means no wheat, either from white flour or whole-wheat flour. This is not being totally gluten-free, just no wheat. This is not easy, as it means no regular bread, pasta, muffins, cookies, or crackers for a few weeks. Find 100% rye crackers, 100% rye bread, rice crackers, quinoa pasta, etc, to get through the two weeks. In case you need a few cookies, almond or coconut macaroons are usually wheat-free. Other food categories that people try skipping to experience some symptomatic improvements are: dairy, eggs, soy and corn.[224]

Finally, give extra support directly to repair the joints. Think about repairing cartilage cells and adding to the cushioning fluid in the joint spaces. The best recommendation is a not-so-well known supplement, a collagen extracted from the sternum bones of chickens, called **biocell collagen**. There is a good amount of research on it, for both osteoarthritis (2 grams per day)[225] and rheumatoid arthritis (40 mg undenatured collagen Type II).[226] People taking it also experience better skin elasticity[227], and stronger hair and nails. My experience is that people will feel the beneficial effects in about 2 weeks. A few people are sometimes allergic to Collagen Type I and Type III, so be a little careful when trying this. If you can handle chicken soup, chances are you'll be okay, though.

You may already have heard about **Glucosamine sulfate** and **Chondroitin sulfate**. These pills sometimes come with **MSM (methylsulfonylmethane)**. MSM adds a nice dose of anti-inflammatory action to the blend. You can use it plain or along with collagen Type II.[228] This plant form of sulfur does not have the risks that aspirin and ibuprofen do. The popular press and medical literature have a variety of opinions on whether Glucosamine-Chondroitin-MSM works or not. I'll say there are a number of quality studies showing efficacy when taken together. It can take 8 weeks of treatment to start getting the repair benefits, so be patient. They don't work as well alone, and if you are obese, they are likely not going to help. The extra weight distresses the joints more than the repair materials can restore the joint surfaces.

One more item you can try that could have some effect in reducing the inflammation and discomfort of rheumatoid arthritis. There are a few small studies that mention the probiotic **Lactobacillus casei**, when taken as a 1 billion colony forming unit supplement each day, can reduce inflammation in rheumatoid arthritis cases.[229]

Energy Healing for Arthritis

You have likely seen television images of elderly Asian people in a public park doing Tai Chi or Chigung exercises. Included the Eastern concept of health preservation is the idea of **Chi** (pronounced "chee"), a subtle bioelectric energy, running from head to toe. When Chi flows, the body maintains better repair function. Many people find modalities that get Chi flowing to be a really good treatment for arthritis. Tai Chi, Chigung, Acupuncture,[230][231] Reflexology, and a Chinese massage technique called Tuina can all help arthritis symptoms quite a bit. Interestingly, a team at Mass General Hospital has described brain lobe changes, as detected by functional MRI's, during acupuncture treatments for knee osteoarthritis.[232] There is a newer modality for getting chi flowing, using brain wave entrainment that is helping reduce arthritis symptoms. Read about **Tong Ren** later in this book.

Nutrition for Metabolic Systems
Growing Immune Cells and Improving Immune Cell Function

A brief story … I was hanging out at a health fair at a local vitamin shoppe a while back with my **The Nutritionist is IN** sign, on a table near the entrance. In cameo appearances at stores like this, people come in, see me and my sign, and ask questions. This helps me keep in touch with what is on the public's mind in the area of nutrition, and I enjoy chatting with the customers, many of whom are impressively well read, thanks in part to internet information.

On this day, a 60-something year-old woman came up to me and asked if the 1000 microgram biotin pills she was holding in her hand would help her grow thicker hair. (1000 mcg is 3.3 times the RDA). I replied that I knew people sometimes grew less hair in a biotin deficiency, and that taking added biotin could sometimes produce more hair. I needed to know a little more about her before I could give a good opinion about the possible usefulness of the biotin she had in her hand. She mentioned that she was already taking B-complex vitamins as part of her supplement regime. (These frequently have a biotin component, so she was unlikely to be deficient.) I suggested that she look into the product called BioSil, a silicon pill that many people do find beneficial for growing stronger nails and thicker hair. She had not heard of this, so she was going to do more reading before she bought it.

As she mentioned that she was taking many supplements, I asked if what she was using included L-glutamine, Coenzyme Q10 and anti-oxidant multivitamins, and she said, "No". I suggested that this basic array would support more general growth and repair in her whole body. I urged her to first take this baseline support, and then in 3 or 4 months see what might be needed for specific parts, like hair and nails. I also asked if she ate a protein food item at breakfast. "No," she replied.

The woman's biotin question points out the mind-set of many people when it comes to nutrition treatments. Their approach is much like Western medicine: what is the symptom, and what pill will treat it? Nutrition therapy is seldom this simple. Nutrition support is essentially environmental therapy: be sure all the essential ingredients are present in correct proportions for the system to run. Here's an example. Since calcium is the major component of bones, at one time people just worried about having plenty of it to be sure bones grew strong. Once the effects of vitamin D on bone calcification became known, adding vitamin D supplements became the standard. There is an important magnesium component to bone structure, so some forward thinking companies add magnesium to their bone support supplement mix. It turns out that strontium and boron are crucial to having strong bones too. Meanwhile, what people are not looking at is whether the body feels like directing all these resources to bones. If there is an excess of inflammation (free radicals coursing through the body), food and supplements won't get to bones; other repair systems will get priority. Osteoporosis will still happen, even in a resource-rich setting. Good diet and smart supplements won't work if the milieu is not right.

As you read in the previous pages, the gut is an ecosystem. Having it in good shape involves multiple items: a variety of food fiber, good bacteria, and, sometimes, certain extra amino acids. Wanting other body parts to grow well too, like hair or nails, can also involve a complex of repair materials. For a nutrition solution, don't just think about a body part and the pill to fix it. Think about broad-spectrum support.

Processing Carbohydrates
Blood Sugar, Insulin Resistance, and Diabetes

In the course of aging, many processing and repair systems in the body function a bit more slowly. Included in the decline is the handling of carbohydrate calories, as managed by the insulin system.[233] Most people, even without some family history of blood sugar issues, will have some decline in insulin signal and receptor function as they age. Added to this could be the shifts in metabolism caused by the inflammation of arthritis, or lung conditions, or intestinal glitches. The result can be that blood sugar levels remain a little higher after meals.

Science Lesson

The body has a system for maintaining a steady supply of blood sugar to the brain, and for distributing the extra sugar from meals to other body parts such as muscles. After you eat pasta, potatoes, apples, and peas digestion breaks down their carbohydrate calories to glucose: the sugar molecule—$C_6H_{12}O_6$—you may have heard about in your school science classes. So the glucose travels in the blood stream and the brain automatically gets a supply. When there is extra sugar in the blood, the pancreas releases some insulin, which tells cells that are next to arteries to open up and let the sugar molecules in. Insulin keeps doors open for about 20 to 30 minutes. After the extra sugar moves into muscles, insulin trails off and the doors close, leaving a crucial baseline amount of sugar to feed the brain. The body wants to provide a steady level of blood glucose to the brain at all times. The diagram below illustrates insulin action.

The term **"diabetes"** literally means "sugar trapped in the blood: not moving into cells." It is a descriptive term. In **Type 1** diabetes, "juvenile onset", something has happened in the pancreas, and suddenly no insulin is produced to do the job of directing sugar into cells. There is also **Type 2** diabetes, "adult onset". In Type 2, there is generally plenty of insulin, but insulin's "move sugar" command is not getting through to cells. Either the insulin message is being ignored, *i.e.* actually "resisted," or the insulin is simply not talking to muscle and other cells well enough. **"Impaired glucose tolerance"** is another term, describing the situation where insulin is sort of working, but sugar clearance from the blood is slower than usual. Type 2 diabetes shows up as higher sugar in the blood of a person generally after age 55 or 60, though some late 40's and early 50's diagnoses occur. A recent trend is that obese 16-year-olds are also getting the diagnosis.

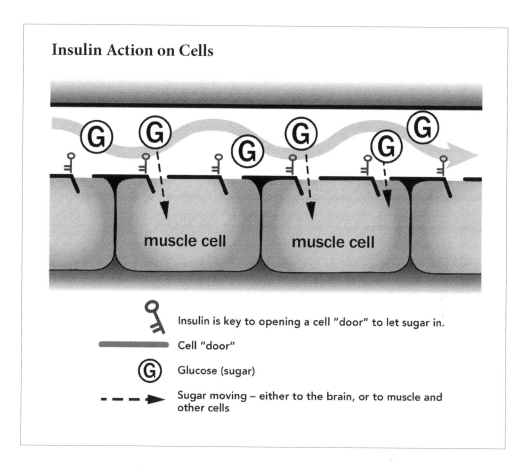

Insulin Action on Cells

muscle cell   muscle cell

Insulin is key to opening a cell "door" to let sugar in.

Cell "door"

Glucose (sugar)

Sugar moving – either to the brain, or to muscle and other cells

Type 2 diabetes: it's not just about the pancreas

When people hear that they have type II diabetes, the language and culture of the medical industrial establishment gives them the impression that they now and forever will have this "disease." The vibe is that they will need medicine to manage this problem the rest of their life! A cautionary flag about this should be raised however.

People need to step back and take another view, separate from the idea that costly prescription medications are the only way to manage diabetes. A better perspective could be that you likely have a significant amount of insulin resistance and your blood sugars are higher than normal, so ask, "Why this insulin resistance now? Are there some parts of me that are stressed, and need repair?"

Type 2 diabetes is a symptom: the problem is usually excess inflammation!

Insulin sluggishness or outright resistance can be provoked by many cellular events around the body. The major underlying mechanism is a response to inflammation.[234] However, there are fuel-processing systems to consider. Many times the body may actually not want sugar to be absorbed into certain places, so that it can be readily used in other body areas. The body may also want to preferentially burn fat when there is too much of it someplace, so it blocks sugar movement. Example, when clogged with too much fat, the liver tries to keep sugar out of its cells, so it "resists" the insulin message that is telling it to absorb the glucose. Eventually, when there is too much insulin resistance over a period of months or years, a diagnosis of diabetes can happen.

Most important: if you have Type 2 diabetes, don't feel as though you have now begun some automatic progression of continuously more complicated medical regimens. Take a step back and do a whole body assessment.

Conditions that Generate Insulin Resistance which are Alterable

1. Food truly is your first medicine

Improving food choices and intake patterns can make a major difference in blood sugars. It is important to point this out because you should save medications for when they are really needed. This approach is good for the whole body. Among the useful elements in fruits and vegetables are substances called polyphenols. Flavones in citrus fruits, and phloridzin in apples are two examples. These compounds improve blood sugar management, and help lower LDL-cholesterol.[235]

In the famous **Diabetes Prevention Trial**[236] the experiment was to see which was better for normalizing blood sugars in people with impaired glucose tolerance. Some people worked on diet and fitness, while others took a drug called Metformin. Not only did diet and exercise work better than drug therapy at normalizing blood sugars, these people even reduced their need for blood pressure and cholesterol therapies for the whole next decade.

My observation is that in the past 10 years or so, as soon as someone has any high blood sugar lab results, they are put on the drug glucophage, also called

Metformin®. A decade or three ago, a doctor would have asked the patient to first try controlling their blood sugar with diet.

2. Are you really eating well?

Food changes alone can make a major difference in glucose metabolism. Eating more red meat, cheese, refined grains, and less wine is the food pattern associated with developing diabetes.[237] Over-eating both fat and carbohydrate calories causes inflammation.[238] Again, inflammation causes poor insulin function. Simply eating less food can begin to reverse diabetes. Making specific food changes also lowers blood sugars. A move to more Mediterranean cuisine is a start toward better health. Taking antioxidant vitamins and switching to olive oil as your only cooking oil can improve sugar processing.[239] A supper of grilled shrimp or scallops, basted in garlic-infused olive oil and served on top of a spinach salad is a prescription for diabetes reversal.

Nutrient imbalances can cause inflammation. An excess of high fructose corn syrup[240] in the diet, or excess fructose in the setting of insufficient magnesium,[241] and even an imbalance in the ratio of calcium to magnesium can all impair the ability of insulin to clear sugar from the blood.[242] **Magnesium** is a complicated nutrient in aging and blood sugar issues. Older intestines may not absorb magnesium as well. Insulin resistance causes disruption in magnesium flow. Low magnesium at the cell level causes more insulin resistance.[243] Remember to eat magnesium foods daily, and get 100 mg or more in your vitamins. Quick quiz: name me three foods that are great sources of magnesium. A delicious diet that removes these stumbling blocks is easy. You know the solution: Paleo-era style cuisine where you have turkey sausage, applesauce, and smoked almonds for breakfast. Include black beans or lentils in your lunch salad, along with your tuna or chicken. Supper is haddock with garlic and capers, plus asparagus anointed with olive oil and lemon juice, plus some smoked red lentils.

3. Exercise and fitness

Whether carrying excess weight or not, starting an exercise program can reverse insulin resistance.[244] Remember, being out of shape, also known as being under-exercised, is 3 times as risky for your health as having a high cholesterol count. Muscle conditioning also affects insulin response and glucose clearance. What can you imagine doing to start getting some conditioning going? Walking 30 minutes has significant positive health benefits. People need to do some upper-body muscle toning activity, too. Most sports stores sell equipment that will help with muscle toning. Using big rubber bands with handles and a wall chart showing how to use them is recommended. You can be "pumping rubber" while watching television.

4. Are you at a healthy weight?

Even if you are carrying just an extra 10 or 15 lbs of body weight, do something to reduce it. Obviously, diet and exercise are the smart place to start. Where you carry your extra pounds has added meaning. Weight in the belly area, versus spread out all over the body means more risk of blood sugar and blood fat problems.[245] This is the apple shape (fat above the waist) versus pear shape (fat below the waist) description. I add the Waist to Hip ratio info here because I hope that you'll really work on improving your numbers if you are at risk.

A higher Waist to Hip ratio is an indication that inflammation levels are likely higher than they should be. Trying to lose belly fat is harder than usual weight reduction. I urge people to get some supplemental support. Supplements include a better-than-average antioxidant vitamin as mentioned previously. Also, take 3 to 4 grams per day fish oils.[246] Frequently, belly fat causes the blood fats

---

Calculate your Waist to Hip ratio.

1. Measure your waist at the belly button, in inches.

2. Measure your hips at the widest part across your butt, in inches.

3. Do the math, or use your computer's calculator:

Waist (in inches)		Hips (in inches)		Waist to Hip ratio
_____	÷	_____	=	_____

4. Check your risk to health complications like diabetes, hypertension, and heart disease

Men	Women	Category
0.95 or below	0.80 or below	Low Risk
0.96 to 1.0	0.81 to 0.85	Moderate Risk
1.0+	0.85+	High Risk

called "triglycerides" to be higher. If concerned about triglycerides, then also take 1 gram per day of either the amino acid called L-carnitine or the one called acetyl L-carnitine[247] for a few months. Supplemental L-carnitine helps liver cells burn fat better. After 2 or 3 months, as weight loss is progressing, just rely on dietary protein to support L-carnitine requirements. Beef has more L-carnitine than do chicken, pork and fish.

This is another reason why I advocate eating grass-fed red meat once a week or so. Grass-fed lamb is available in many stores, like Trader Joe's. FYI, it is L-carnitine that provides the "gamey" taste in meats like lamb; mutton (adult sheep) is the best dietary source. That's not a popular food these days in the USA anyway.

Body Mass Index is another calculation for assessing weight status. It is weight in kilograms, divided by height in meters, squared. [example: 70 kg divided by (1.70m)2 = 24.2]. A BMI >25 and <30 is "over-weight"; a BMI greater than 30 means obesity. The obese label certainly carries a lot of emotion with it. I mention the term here just for a point of science, or medical fact. Significant excess fat creates conditions that impair glucose processing. Again, it is all about inflammation. Fat cells, especially those in the belly area send out distress signals that can cause insulin resistance. Think about it. You are a fat cell, you don't want to get any bigger; next time someone is trying to deliver excess sugars for you to store as fat, you're going to resist the message. It is also about the physics. Fat is taking up space and as a result is blocking insulin's access to receptors on cell surfaces.

Extra fat in the gut area often accompanies a condition called "fatty liver." A liver that is choking on excess fat will also send out a signal to resist the efforts of insulin to send in more sugar that will turn to fat.[248] As mentioned above, fish oils and L-carnitine plus fewer calories are the best remedial strategy for unclogging a fatty liver.

I promote authentic nutrition first, and diabetes medicines second. Weight gain is a common side effect of diabetes treatment. Extra fat weight gets in the way of good blood sugar control. Why does the weight gain happen? The medicines are forcing sugar into liver and fat cells, making them accumulate fat they often didn't want to have in the first place. In the case of the thiazolidinedione drugs, (examples: Avandia® and Actos®), this therapy seems to increase risk of heart attacks,[249] and some cancers.[250] You can feel very comfortable taking a few extra caveman-era nutrients and not raise your risk of heart disease or cancer. Give serious thoughts to a smart food plan, plus omega-3 EPA/DHA fish oils, and L-carnitine as your first therapy for blood sugar issues. Again, start with nutrients to fix sugar metabolism; resort to medicine later, if needed.

5. Key nutrients that help insulin work

Let's talk about some more nutrients that may be deficient and which might be why people develop blood sugar problems. **Vitamin D** is high on the list. Something about having decent vitamin D levels keeps sugar moving better.[251] You want to know where your vitamin D levels are for many reasons, anyhow. **Chromium**, a mineral needed in just trace amounts, is crucial to carbohydrate metabolism. Many health food stores and nutrition books will recommend it for diabetes care. I am conservative on this one. You can get 100 to 200 micrograms of chromium per day in a smart vitamin supplement, and that is a sufficient dose.[252] Taking 400 micrograms chromium per day for three months has a bit of usefulness for lowering fasting sugars.[253] Higher doses over time could disrupt the absorption of other trace minerals, like copper, and the cause of such deficiencies would be hard to detect. There is one added twist to the chromium story: a neutraceutical company combined the amino acid cysteine, plus the vitamin niacin, with a chromium pill. The combo did show a reversal of insulin resistance and reduction in inflammation markers.[254] Remember, you read about cysteine supporting the antioxidant enzyme glutathione back in the lung section of this book. As I said before, Type 2 diabetes is frequently an excess inflammation problem. Read more about glutathione in the next section about glutamine.

Nutrients that are part of cell construction are subtle modulators of glucose metabolism. Let's look at EPA/DHA omega-3 fats. All cell membranes are made up of the fat molecules we eat. A cell can survive on corn oil or lard in its structure but it will function better when it has a certain amount of EPA/DHA fat in its membrane architecture. In this case, the insulin message is more effective when there are EPA/DHA molecules in the muscle and liver cell membranes.[255] A deficiency of EPA/DHA omega-3 fats is hard to detect .

Certain amino acids present in muscle cell surface proteins also help carbohydrate processing. **L-glutamine** is a key player here. It helps keep muscles in their optimum state of repair, so that insulin receptors are in good shape too.[256] Glutamine also has a role in improving insulin signaling.[257] It supports the glutathione antioxidant enzyme too.

The amino acid Arginine helps glucose handling as well.[258][259] At this time I don't usually recommend it as a supplement; I am waiting for some safety studies to be completed. Use L-glutamine first.

L-glutamine is extra special

I find the amino acid L-glutamine a very useful supplement for many patients, especially those with blood sugar problems. People with diabetes or insulin resistance frequently have mood problems. The hard part to figure out is which came first, the mood problem or the diabetes.[260] A person's mood drop can be a result of worrying over food management and blood sugar testing. Hypoglycemic events wear people down emotionally too. It can be lifestyle elements, such as less exercise or less nutritious eating. Depression can cause the insulin resistance.

When in doubt, first vote biology, then psychology. Common to both diabetes and depression is a higher than usual amount of inflammation in the neuro-endocrine systems, plus a failure of the immune system to clean up enough.[261] A deeper analysis of brain metabolism in people with diabetes and depression shows that their brains are low in L-glutamine.[262] There are no intervention trials to improve levels in diabetics yet though. However, studies of people who are receiving L-glutamine supplementation as part of a bone marrow transplant treatment for cancer show improvement in mood.[263]

Trying L-glutamine simply involves taking a simple one teaspoon dose of powder, (4.5 grams) each morning. The only people who should not take extra glutamine are people on a protein-restricted diet due to their advanced liver or kidney disease. Pregnant women should not take glutamine either, but then again, that is not a likely event for the primary audience of this book. One warning, glutamine often makes people feel the buzz of caffeine more intensely. You may need to have part decaf in your morning coffee. Anyone who has SIBO, small intestine bacterial overgrowth, may want to start with just a ½ teaspoon dose for a few days.

6. Hormones and blood sugar management

Hormones also have a big influence on sugar metabolism. As part of reversing sugar processing problems, you might consider knowing what your hormone levels are. For men, **low testosterone** levels can mean more blood sugar issues.[264] An extreme example of low testosterone occurs in men on hormone suppressive therapy as part of their prostate cancer treatment. They are at much higher risk for diabetes.[265] Men may want to know their "total" and "free" testosterone levels when working on reversing insulin resistance. If testosterone levels are low, first look at some lifestyle issues for getting the body's own systems working naturally. Excessive alcohol intake can reduce testosterone levels.[266] Not getting an adequate amount of sleep also lowers testosterone.[267]

There are several ways to raise testosterone levels. A moderate weight lifting exercise program raises testosterone levels in men in both their early 20's and in their late 40's.[268][269] The increase in testosterone production that can come from lifting weights does diminish with age, but there is still some benefit.[270] If considering a therapy to raise testosterone, look into Eastern medicine treatments first, like acupuncture or Tong Ren. There are prescription testosterone gels to try as well. Testim® is the gel that seems to be most recommended by the best-informed endocrine doctors around Boston. Gels can be expensive. You could learn to give yourself weekly hormone injections too at a fraction of the cost. A fantastic resource for testosterone replacement information is www.excelmale.com. Men with prostate health issues, like elevated PSA, should not go on testosterone. This warning is getting re-examined by some savvy docs in Boston, like Abe Morgantaler.[271] Be prepared that when you ask your doctor to consider testosterone replacement therapy for you, there will likely be resistance. It is a topic that needs updating in the medical literature. The journal *Endocrine* published an article: *Testosterone in men with hypogonadism and high cardiovascular risk, Pros.*[272] in 2015. It essentially states that benefits outweigh any risks.

Women need adequate levels of DHEA (dehydroepiandrosterone) and testosterone as well.[273] It matters to the health of their bones, muscles, and mood. The body uses DHEA to make testosterone and estrogen. Women worrying about blood sugar clearance may want to know blood levels of both DHEA and testosterone. No need for prescription testosterone gel for women. DHEA supplements are inexpensive and have less risk of over-doing it. There is quite an extensive research literature on the use of DHEA supplements in post-menopausal women, and a modest one in men. In one study in a 2004 Journal of American Med Assoc. DHEA supplements helped lower abdominal fat in 56 people, average age 71.[274] In a 2006 paper in The New England Journal of Medicine, DHEA or testosterone didn't affect body fat in 83 elderly people. There is no mention of belly fat however. There are some reports of slight improvement in bone mineralization. With blood monitoring of DHEA levels, it is safe.[275] Monitor testosterone levels as well. Excess testosterone is not good, obviously. All in all, DHEA seems to offer only a small possible payoff in helping blood sugar management, and bone mineralization, but people need to know about it. There has been a modest number of patients who have benefited from it.

7. Take care of bones to help blood sugars

Science does not have a full picture on how and why bones play a role in regulating glucose metabolism and insulin messaging. There seem to be some chemical signals that run between fat cells, bone cells and the insulin-producing beta cells of the pancreas.[276] You just want to be sure your bones are doing their best repair work. As you have read in the bone health section, don't rely on drugs for bone health; instead, be authentically nourished. Have plenty of nutrients on hand, in the right amounts, including vitamin D, and magnesium and vitamin K2, plus the trace minerals boron and strontium.

8. Know Your C-Reactive Protein (CRP) Level

C-Reactive Protein (CRP) is often measured as a way to check if someone with borderline high cholesterol is at more risk for heart disease. CRP measures inflammation. Higher CRP will suggest that circulating cholesterol is more likely to cause arterial narrowing. Meanwhile, in the diabetes arena, as CRP goes higher, insulin resistance also rises.[277] A higher CRP is an indication that the body is working on repairing something, but is missing some key nutrients. For example, 2 to 3 mg/day of vitamin B6 is the suggested intake for seniors. In healthy aging less than 10% of people will be found to have low levels of B6 at that intake level. However, in a setting of high CRP, 50% of people will be found to be low in B6 according to a study from the USDA Nutrition and Aging Center in Boston.[278] Once again, here is an indication that some extra B-complex vitamins are a good idea for older people, even in the setting of a good diet. As mentioned before, higher CRP relates to faster brain aging too. All in all, if higher CRP persists, get some help figuring out what body parts are not successfully repairing due to inadequate nutrients, including all B vitamins,[279] vitamin D, [280] and selenium.[281]

Diabetes Diet Therapy

Antioxidant-rich diet, plus an antioxidant vitamin

You now know that excess inflammation is a big factor causing insulin resistance. With more antioxidants in your diet you will lower your risk for, and the incidence of, insulin resistance.[282] A quality diet is potent for reducing inflammation and quickly reversing insulin resistance. Some added nutrients, like vitamin C and vitamin E alone or in combination, add some potency to an anti-diabetic scheme.[283][284][285] This makes the Life Extension Foundation multivitamin product called **Two Per Day Tablets** an excellent choice in initial diabetic diet support.

Animal studies show that antioxidants are supporting the glutathione (antioxidant) enzyme, and something called Hepatic Insulin Sensitizing Substance (HISS).[286] This helps insulin effectively connect to muscles. HISS is expressed in larger amounts after a meal (with some protein), versus after a snack, and it accounts for 50% of the insulin's ability to deliver its message.[287] While this sounds like a lot of science, I mention it simply as a way to emphasize how dynamic food really is in body processes. Recently, the USDA published the results of a study where the researchers were providing a fruit-fiber-antioxidant bar to people twice a week, for just 2 weeks. They reported how glutathione levels started to rise, and inflammation started to go down. It was too short a time to alter insulin function in the study, but when 4 doses of a nutritious snack bar eaten over two weeks are reducing whole-body inflammation, this is proof that nutrition is powerful.[288]

More Metabolic Support Supplements to Help the Diabetic Diet

Another dynamic supplement to know about, for helping reverse insulin resistance, is the amino acid **L-carnitine**.[289] As I mentioned a few pages back, cells are sometimes clogged with fat, and become insulin-resistant in order to clear out the fat. L-carnitine facilitates fat burning in liver and muscle cells. Unburned fat fragments that are hanging around cells cause irritation. Again, the irritation causes release of the cytokine (chemical messenger) Tumor Necrosis Factor *alpha* (TNFa) which is antagonistic to insulin action.

One more supplement I'll mention here is **alpha lipoic acid**. It is an antioxidant substance that supports better glutathione levels.[290] You have read enough now to know this will help insulin action. Being a comprehensive antioxidant, it works to lower the risk of nerve and vascular complications caused by high sugar and insulin.[291]

The added benefit of alpha lipoic acid here is that it also helps muscles absorb sugar without needing as much insulin as usual. Lower insulin messaging means fewer "build fat" and "make hungry" messages. *Glucophage* (Metformin®) is generally the first drug given to people to manage sugar. A number of people get nausea and other gut side effects from it for several months. I prefer that people try alpha lipoic acid first.

Excess sugar hanging around the blood stream is, itself, an irritant. As you now appreciate, irritation plays out as inflammation. Irritation can raise the rate of sticky LDL-cholesterol clogging arteries. The inflammation also bothers cells in arteries in another way. Arteries get "expand-and-contract" signals for managing blood flow. When an expansion signal happens, but the blood vessels suddenly contract instead. This is called "endothelial dysfunction". It can cause very high blood pressure. Endothelial dysfunction is something to worry about in people with blood sugar problems and it is one mechanism for higher risk for heart failure. Nutrition can come to the rescue of course. The supplement **Coenzyme Q10, 200mg a day** prevents endothelial dysfunction in people with type 2 diabetes.[292] After urging use of a good multivitamin, I suggest 100mg Co Q10 every day for anyone over 50 wanting to maintain good health. The dose may be higher in certain medical situations.

Diabetes Medications

At some point in diabetes care, you may get started on medicines. You commonly begin with Metformin® (glucophage), as a pill to help lower sugar. It tries to make insulin receptors be more sensitive. The next drugs used to lower sugar are glipizide (Glucotrol®), or glyburide (Micronase® and Diabeta®). These squeeze more insulin out of pancreatic cells, often causing them to run out of the ability to produce insulin sooner, putting people on a faster course to needing insulin injections. The next step in pills to manage sugars has been the "glitazone" drugs. It turns out that these convey added heart attack and bladder cancer risks so their use is now curtailed. Other pills and injected drugs are coming on the market; each has benefits, but also side effects and risks, like thyroid cancer or more foot and toe amputations.[293] Often, the last resort is injected insulin. Modern insulin therapy is getting easier, with the advent of slow acting, once-a-day injections with names like Levemir® and Lantus®. Remember, though, being on injections becomes a more complex self-care event.

You need to be on a consistent meal and snack regimen, or sugars can drop too low. Diabetes is not an easy condition to treat. No pill is as potent as a good diet and exercise are. Get help with the diet if you are struggling to eat as well as you need to. Doing your homework in the beginning will pay big dividends in fewer complications later.

Details of the Diet for Insulin Resistance

Now imagine the blood sugar curve caused by what you eat …

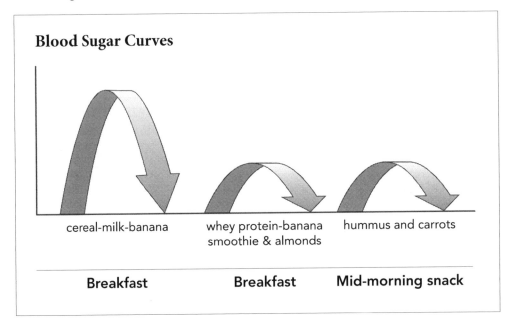

Let's start with terminology. "Glycemic index" refers to how quickly a dose of some sweet or carbohydrate food will raise blood sugar levels. Next, "glycemic load" refers to the volume of blood sugar in circulation after you eat. The bigger the load, the bigger the insulin response will need to be. Insulin makes people feel hungrier and have more sugar cravings. As you look at the arrows above, you can imagine a big dose of carbs that rise in a hurry can strain your insulin system more than the two smaller loads.

Diet plans taught to diabetics are still rife with poor advice. Anyone having a diabetic breakfast composed of cereal, milk and banana is tragically misled. All three foods digest to become blood sugar, which then requires an insulin response. The triple carb breakfast bowl is absurd. Having the Paleolithic (protein-fruit-nut) breakfast is simply a much lower glucose challenge to the system, plus it supports better insulin messaging action.

Keeping insulin expression lower has many benefits. Remember, insulin makes people hungry. Many people with diabetes complain of constant sugar cravings all day. It is often some wrong breakfast advice for a diabetic that makes them hungry all day!

Insulin Messages

1. Move sugar into cells

2. Build fat

3. Retain sodium (raising blood pressure)

4. Make hungry / crave sweets

When it comes to lunch and dinner, remember, meals with lean proteins and legumes, plus huge amounts of vegetables are therapeutic. Among protein choices at meals include fish with omega-3 fats often.[294] Again, make an effort to eat magnesium-rich foods. In a study that followed the diet habits of about 4,500 healthy 30-year-olds for 20 years, lower magnesium intake was one of the prime habits of people who developed diabetes![295]

Refer back to the Sample Food Plans in Part 3 of this book to assemble low glycemic meals and snacks.

You could also approach your plate composition with an eye toward geometry. Assemble foods on your plate with the configurations you see in the next few pages of diagrams.

Plate Composition For Sugar Control

Breakfast

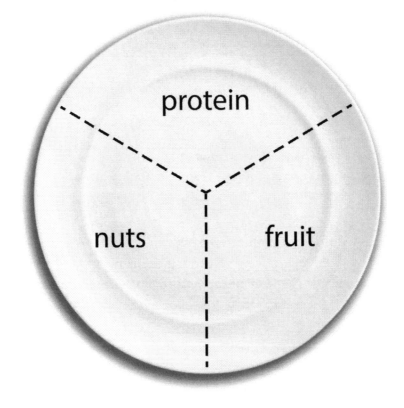

protein

nuts

fruit

Morning Snack

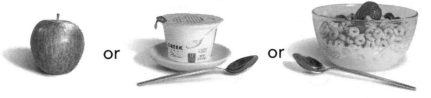

fruit   or   Greek yogurt   or   cereal or starch

Plate Composition For Sugar Control

Lunch

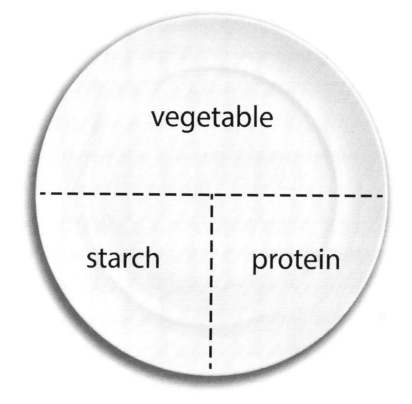

vegetable

starch | protein

Afternoon Snack

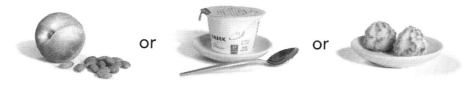

or   or

A fruit and a
handful of nuts

Greek yogurt

macaroons

*Nuts & berries are the ideal, but other days
it may be a yogurt or 2 cookies.*

Plate Composition For Sugar Control

Dinner

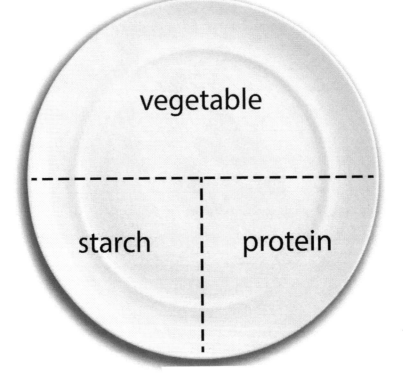

vegetable

starch | protein

Evening Snack

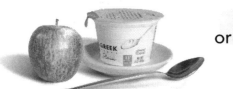

or

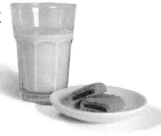

fruit & yogurt

milk and
2 fig newtons

Usually fruit and yogurt; occasionally, milk and 2 cookies.

Guide to Groceries

The extra–fierce foods are in **bold type**. These are items that have been mentioned in various sections throughout the book.

REPAIR FOODS: **PROTEIN**

Blue fish
Cod
Flounder
Haddock
Herring
Lobster
Salmon
Sardines
Shrimp
Scallops
Trout
Tuna

Whey protein powder
No fat/low-fat cottage
   cheese
Egg whites/ EggBeaters
Veggie burger
Turkey breast
Turkey ham
Turkey sausage
Chicken breast
Chicken legs
Chicken thighs
Pork chop

Pork tenderloin
Lite/low-fat cheeses
Omega-3 eggs

Grass-fed is best:
Lamb chops
Lean beef
Cheese, especially
   goat & sheep

Collagen peptides

CALCIUM FOODS

Almond milk
Low fat/skim milk

Dark greens
Yogurt

Bone Repair
Algae sources
www.Algaecal.com

ANTIOXIDANT & IMMUNE SYSTEM FOODS: **VEGETABLES**

Asparagus
Bok choy
Broccoli
Brussels sprouts
Cabbage
Carrots
Cauliflower
Celery
Collard greens
Cucumbers
Dandelion greens

Dark green lettuce
Eggplant
Green/yellow beans
Green/red/hot peppers
Kale
Mushrooms
Mustard greens
Okra
Onions
Parsley
Parsnips

Pea pods
Purslane
Spinach
Summer squash
Swiss chard
Tomatoes
Tomato sauce
Winter squash
Zucchini squash

—Continued on next page

Guide to Groceries

ANTIOXIDANT & IMMUNE SYSTEM FOODS: **FRUITS**

It's better to eat solid fruit than drink juices.

Apples
Applesauce
Apricots
Bananas
Blackberries
Blueberries
Cantaloupe
Clementines
Grapefruit
Honeydew
Kiwis
Lychee
Mangos
Nectarines
Oranges

Papaya
Peaches
Pears
Pineapple
Plums
Pomegranate
Raspberries
Red grapes
Strawberries
Watermelon

Dried fruit (extra sweet)
Dates
Figs
Raisins
Cran-raisins

4 oz juices
Apricot nectar
Grape juice
Grapefruit juice
Orange juice
Pineapple juice
Red pomegranate
    juice

ENERGY FOODS: **STARCHES & CARBOHYDRATES**

Black beans
Black-eyed peas
Chickpeas
Hummus
Lentils
Lima beans
Navy beans
Pinto beans
Red kidney beans
Sweet potatoes
White kidney beans
Yams

100% Rye bread

Barley
Buckwheat
Cheerios
Corn
Corn tortillas
Millet
Oat Bran
Oatmeal
Peas
Plantain
Potatoes
Quinoa
Rice

Careful
Bagels
Cakes
Candy
Cookies
Muffins
Noodles
Pancakes
Saltines
Spaghetti
Waffles
White bread
Whole wheat bread

—Continued on next page

Guide to Groceries

ENERGY FOODS: **FATS & OILS**

Almonds	**Chia seeds**	*Be modest*
Brazil nuts	**Ground flax seeds**	Butter (grass fed is
Cashews	Hemp seeds	nice)
Hazelnuts	Pepitas	Lard
Macadamia nuts	Pumpkin seeds	
Peanuts	Sesame seeds	*Avoid*
Pecans	Sunflower seeds	Canola oil
Pine nuts		Corn oil
Pistachio nuts	Avocado	Cotton seed oil
Soy nuts	Coconut oil	Cream cheese
Walnuts	**Olives**	Fried fast foods
	Olive oil	Safflower oil
	Peanut oil	Stick margarine
		Vegetable oil

Reversing Diabetic Complications: Neuropathy

Diabetic neuropathy is the term that describes the numbness, burning, and pain in hands or feet that happens to people with blood sugar management problems. Some people with diabetes genes in the family start to develop neuropathy even before they have blood sugar problems. The "thrift gene" that makes people at higher risk for diabetes also causes a fat processing glitch. The common fat linolenic acid (LA) that people get in corn oil and vegetable oil does not get converted to gamma linolenic acid (GLA) adequately.[296]

There are multiple consequences to having low GLA levels in the body then.

- Cholesterol levels rise.

- Triglyceride levels rise.

- HDL (good) cholesterol levels drop.

- Skin becomes dry: cracks happen on the ends of thumbs and fingers.

- Nerve cells don't repair and start to give a burning feeling, then numbness: neuropathy.

Quite simply, a little known reason for diabetic neuropathy is the deficiency of the GLA type of fat.[297] The American diet can be low in it as people eat mostly processed oils. Most medical providers are unaware of the genetic issues about GLA in Type 2 diabetes.

Taking GLA as the supplement Evening Primrose Oil frequently reduces neuropathy. Try taking 2.0 to 2.6 grams per day of Evening Primrose oil for 3 months to see how nerves feel. As a food source of GLA, some people use 1 to 2 tablespoons a day of "cold-pressed sunflower seed oil." This works well but finding a local source for it is tough. Borage oil is also a popular suggestion for GLA. I do not recommend borage oil as a supplement, because other chemical compounds in borage oil cause "vasoconstriction," which is a shrinking of blood flow in capillaries. This is not an effect you want as a person with diabetes. Primrose oil supplements do not interfere with any medications.

Neuropathy can also occur because of metabolic debris, like excessive free radicals, which can impede circulation. A supplement that is a potent antioxidant that seems to improve circulation in feet is the antioxidant Alpha Lipoic Acid (ALA).[298] This actually ends up as a "grow more capillaries"(mini-arteries) message in the body. It works in people with painful neuropathy in their feet. Take 300 mg of Alpha Lipoic Acid, twice a day. **Warning:** blood sugar management medicine doses will likely need adjusting to lower levels when you take ALA. As you read in the earlier section, alpha lipoic acid helps muscles absorb sugar better. Try alpha lipoic acid for 2 months to test its benefit for you. Use it for a few more months if you are getting some positive results.

Benfotiamine for Diabetic Neuropathy

One more nutrition supplement known to reverse diabetic neuropathy is benfotiamine. This is a fat-soluble form of Thiamine, which is vitamin B1. Trials in which 300 mg doses were taken twice a day show better results than one 600 mg dose a day.[299] Try it for 1 to 2 months and see how you feel; if it is working, keep going for a few more months to get maximum benefit.

Being Trapped in Too Many Diabetes Medicines

I see pharmaceutical company ads on TV, featuring very overweight female celebrities, praising the diabetes drugs that are keeping their sugar under control. However, they are likely people trapped in their fatness courtesy of the drugs they are pitching. These are affluent people, who are getting the best medical care money can buy. What they are not receiving is smart, functional medicine-type nutritional care. Frequently, a change in diet, accompanied by some added vitamins, permits lowering amounts of medication or even then discontinuing some. Yes, it may be swapping some pills for others, but the benefit is that vitamins don't have side effects or cause health risks.

An example of Alpha Lipoic Acid, Glutamine and other supplements improving blood sugar clearance and reducing insulin needs.

Here's a good example of how eating a better diet and taking nutrition supplements helped an age 50-something woman who was about 100 pounds overweight. For her diabetes, she was taking 85 units of Lantus® insulin each evening. An average Lantus® dose is 20 to 30 units. She was also using fast acting insulin at each meal, adjusting her insulin dose to what her blood sugars were just before eating. She was frustrated that she could not lose weight, no matter how little she ate. She was taking 40 mg of Lipitor® a day to manage her cholesterol. Her ankles were generally swollen with fluid, as her heart was not pumping strongly enough, so she was also taking furosemide (Lasix®), a fluid reduction pill, with just modest benefit for her. Her feet and legs were puffy and sore most every day.

Her frustrations about not being able to lose weight, and having painful swollen ankles made her miserable. She was not all that hungry, and she agreed to eat no starches for a few weeks: no bread, rice, pasta, crackers or cereal. Her only carbs were 3 to 4 small pieces of fruit a day (50 calories each), and the carbohydrate calories found in broccoli, spinach, cauliflower and other vegetables (15 to 40 carbohydrate calories per cup,) eaten two or three times a day. She started out on the caveperson breakfast: cottage cheese, small apple and 15 to 20 almonds. Lunch was a huge raw salad, plus salmon or other fish. Snack was a kiwi or dish of berries, plus a handful of walnuts or cashews or 2 ounces string cheese. Supper, 2 cups of cooked broccoli, spinach, cauliflower or other low calorie vegetables plus 6 to 8 ounces chicken or lean meat. She ate two evening snacks, one was a low calorie yogurt, and the other was more berries or a Clementine.

The "build fat" message from 85 units of insulin is why she was not able to lose weight. Fat cells will only open up and spill their energy to supply fuel in the absence of insulin messaging. I prescribed 300mg Alpha Lipoic Acid, one at breakfast, and one at dinner. This was to help cells absorb sugar without needing so much insulin. With the action of the lipoic acid, and the lower carbohydrate volume in meals, I warned her to be careful about taking too much insulin. Within a day, she no longer needed her fast-acting insulin at meals. Her sugars were lower. Within 10 days, her doctor was lowering her Lantus® dose to 55 units!

Time to address the fluid in the ankles too. Remember, Lipitor® lowers Co Q10 (heart fuel) levels. I asked her to take 100 mg Coenzyme Q10, twice a day for a month, and then to taper to once a day. This gave her heart more energy to better pump fluid out of her legs. You may remember that insulin has a "retain sodium" message (by way of its effect on the hormone aldosterone in the kidney). On the no-starches food plan, there was less insulin around. On the higher vegetable and correct fruits diet, she was getting more potassium, which also pushes sodium out of her body, so her retained fluid levels were dropping. Her ankles were less swollen within a week. Now she was also able to lower her Lasix® dose. Within 2 weeks, she was down by almost 20 lbs. Yes, this was almost all fluid-weight, but it was a huge psychological boost to someone who was feeling so trapped in her weight.

She was delighted to no longer have painful, swollen ankles every day. She was psyched to stay on the quite limited food plan, thanks to experiencing these dynamic positive results. After a month, her system was working better, so she could "cheat" and dip her vegetables in some hummus a few times a week, at lunch.

She also used 500 mg L-carnitine twice a day, to be sure her liver could burn fat well. She took L-glutamine at 5 grams a day to assure optimum insulin messaging in her cells. The regime worked very well. She lost 100 lbs. in about 9 months.

The list of supplements she used at the start:

- Two Per Day Multivitamin Tablets (by Life Extension Foundation), 2/day
- Alpha Lipoic Acid 300 mg pills, 2/day
- Coenzyme Q10 100 mg pill, 2/day
- L-carnitine 500 mg tablet, 2/day
- L-glutamine, powder, 1 teaspoon/day

The point to emphasize here is that her medicines were managing symptoms, like high blood sugar and swollen ankles, but messing up her metabolism. She was willing to change her diet, and take some more nutritional supplement pills for a few months to get her system functioning better. Her "disease" status changed radically. She could reduce the medicines that were in the way of her improving her health. Luckily she had a physician who was willing to work with her, letting her use diet and nutrient supplements. He reduced her meds progressively. Too many medical providers dismiss this nutritional approach to medical care as ineffective, even though they have not experienced it in action. Again, she had a wonderfully open-minded doc.

Fending Off Colds, the Flu, and Pneumonias plus Taming Auto-immune Diseases

As we age, colds seem to last longer and feel more debilitating. In my office, people often mention how their current cold or bronchitis has been lingering for 6 weeks or more. In a way, this demonstrates how the body does repair work more slowly as people age, but 6 weeks is just too long. You can heal faster but you need to know how to support the key players in your immune system.

Science Lesson
How the Immune System Operates

The Innate Immune System
There are immune cells that circulate around the body that have an especially good ability to detect any cells that are "non-self"... which includes germs, viruses, bad genetic material, and the odd cells that could become cancers. The assorted immune cells that are these frontline soldiers constitute the "innate immune system." This system is good for fast responses to germs, mold, viruses, etc., but not especially good at waging huge battles. They will call in more assistance when they need to. Natural Killer (NK) cells are an important component of both the innate immune system and the body's total antiviral effort. Their vigor seems to decline with age.[300] To what extent the decline is inevitable is simply not known. No research has yet described the mechanism of aging for these cells. Meanwhile, NK cells are sensitive to nutrient status. Coenzyme Q10 is important fuel for NK cells. You read previously, that Coenzyme Q10 production starts to decline after age 20, and this can take on clinical significance by age 50. No investigations yet show what the usual NK cell energy status at age 60 or 70 is though. But by age 90 the energy deficit is clear.[301] Investigations do describe a specific immune cell's response pattern in some remarkably healthy older people, but much work remains on how to nurture this in other people.[302]

Adequate levels of the antioxidant enzyme Glutathione is crucial to growing more Natural Killer cells. Oxidative stress from a cold or bronchitis or from inadequate levels of antioxidants in the diet, results in lower glutathione levels. This means the very system that is supposed to squelch a cold or the flu will be struggling to grow enough immune cell troops to fight the invading germs. We know that L-glutamine helps physically stressed athletes maintain better NK cell levels.[303] Supplemental L-glutamine raises glutathione levels and this may be one of the mechanisms accounting for how it helps cells stave off the growth of breast cancer cells.[304] You should also know that many mushrooms, both as food and as extracts, have tremendous Natural Killer cell and all immune system support properties.[305] Instead of green beans or cauliflower as the vegetable on your dinner plate, think about a cup of crimini, button, or shitake mushrooms on your plate, sautéed in olive oil and garlic of course.

The Acquired Immune System

Once innate immune cells, especially NK cells, have engaged foreign cells, they send signals to the "acquired immune system" to do much of the work of squelching the infectious intruders. The acquired immune system is able to make highly specific cells to fight germs, viruses, etc. That is its forte. It makes custom cells, and lots of them. The customizing processes are known as the TH1 and TH2 responses.[306] It is pictured below. Immune cells start out as TH0 cells with no particular design. There are chemical messengers called "cytokines" (many of them released from the NK cells) that tell the immune system to make certain kinds of cells. The cytokines Interleukin 1 (IL1) and Interleukin 2, (IL2) and Interferon direct activity of the TH1 response. Think of this as the launching of PAC man-like cells, technically Cytotoxic T Lymphocytes (CTL's). CTL's attack viruses like the common cold, the flu, or even HIV and Hepatitis C. The ache you feel from the flu is caused by the Interleukin 2 cytokine circulating in the body.

Medical treatment can sometimes involve Interleukin 2 injections to boost immune activity.[307] Interestingly, the amino acid L-glutamine that we talked about in gut cell support and in muscle repair can help IL2 activity be more competent.[308]

If or when the TH1 system doesn't totally conquer the invading germs, or sometimes to finish clearing an infection, the TH2 system comes into play by making antibodies.

The TH1 response relies on a supply of many nutrients. It is particularly dependent on adequate amounts of zinc, selenium, and glutathione. An

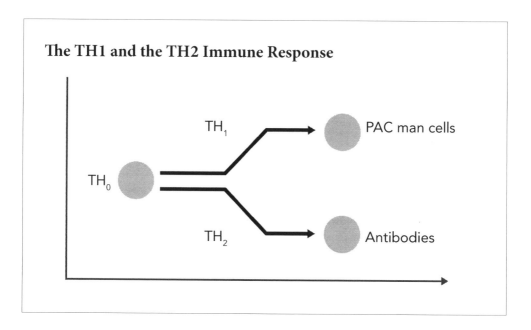

The TH1 and the TH2 Immune Response

important concept is that if the TH1 cell system runs low in zinc, selenium or glutathione, there is a shift to the TH2 (antibody) response.

The TH2 response is directed by cytokines like Interleukin 4 (IL4), Interleukin 5 (IL5), and Interleukin 6 (IL6). These cytokines cause more disturbances in metabolism, and are linked to more damage to human tissue. They rally many more immune cells to charge into an infected area. For example, for Crohn's disease, more IL6 is present in gut tissue. The damage is simply a result of too many immune cells crowding some local tissue.

When people have autoimmune diseases, like rheumatoid arthritis, the "flare ups" are associated with more TH2 response. One way to prevent flare-ups of autoimmune conditions is to keep the TH1 response system well nourished so that the more dynamic TH2 activity is not triggered.

The innate and acquired immune systems rely on many nutrients to operate at their best. Zinc and selenium are two nutrients frequently deficient in older people.[309] This is one of the reasons I advocate taking multivitamins. Check for 15mg of zinc, and 100mcg selenium in yours.

Vitamin C and vitamin E are the main antioxidants fighting free radicals. If they can't handle the volume of free radicals a person is experiencing, then glutathione has to take over squelching free radicals. You already know that glutathione is necessary for producing new NK cells, let me also emphasize that it matters to proper acquired immune cell (CTL) responses too. These Packman-like cells of the TH1 response may not respond adequately if they don't have enough vitamin C or zinc or fruits and vegetables in the diet. The consequence is that not only will a cold or bronchitis linger much longer, but a flare-up of an autoimmune condition like colitis or rheumatoid arthritis can occur when the TH1 system is undernourished.

The Aging Immune System

Why the immune system is less vigorous as people age is a complex story. At the heart of the matter is a less dynamic immune response to germs.[310] As mentioned before, cytokines are the junior hormone-like substances that direct activities of the immune system. In aging, it seems that the cytokines that generate best TH1 response are lagging, and more autoimmune TH2 events are happening. As I mentioned, this TH1 system is quite sensitive to nutritional status, especially with respect to zinc, selenium, and glutathione.[311] The system is also sensitive to DHEA, the adrenal hormone we were discussing in relation to insulin issues in diabetes.[312] Not all the causes of the less vigorous immune response are known yet but one concept to know is "inflamm-aging."[313] The concept is that the body is slow to clean up free radicals as people age so there is more inflammation and this hampers immune cell function. The more antioxidant-rich fruit and vegetables in the diet, the less inflammation people have. Some added vitamin C and vitamin E as supplements play out here too.[314]

Mentioning all the details of the immune system here is to drive home significant points. Maintaining exceptional nutrient intake supports the immune system far more than any drug could. People are inappropriately lulled into a sense of tranquility or safety by things like flu shots.

The true statistics are that the flu vaccine is not that potent for seniors.

The focus on flu shots is something that is troublesome. A hidden fact you may find of interest: in the period from 1980 to 2001, the number of elderly getting flu shots has gone from 15% to 65% of the population, yet there has been no decline in death rate from the flu.[315] This and similar studies are controversial, but the premise remains; don't automatically trust some medicines. Have a plan to take good care of yourself. More mysterious afflictions will be on the horizon, like swine flu and bird flu. Interestingly, there are some studies out of Canada showing that people who received the 2008 – 2009 trivalent flu vaccine became more susceptible to getting the H1N1 swine flu when it came along.[316] Also noteworthy, the anti-flu medicine Tamiflu is already showing signs of becoming ineffective.[317] The more important medical fact is that the pneumonia that sets in after the flu is what causes the most sickness and mortality. Nutrition has a big impact here.

You already know about taking better care of your systems to reduce risk of lung and other troubles. It starts with your gut flora population to help your lungs stay more immune competent against the pneumonia. There are vitamins for immune support, and we've discussed 200iu of vitamin E to help the flu shot be more effective for those of you who get one.

In order to reduce sick time from a cold, or to keep a cold from progressing to bronchitis or pneumonia, look at the list of supplements below, and consider using them during the high risk winter months. Each item, the vitamins, the glutamine, the cysteine, has clinical data to support its use in diminishing the risk or duration of a viral illness. Sadly, there is not yet a trial showing the likely greater efficacy when combined as a therapy.

Daily Supplements to Prepare for Coping With Colds and Flu

1. **Multivitamin** that contains
   10X the RDA for B-complex
   100 mg to 200 mg vitamin C
   100 units to 200 units vitamin E
   100 mcg to 200 mcg selenium
   15-30 mg zinc

   Examples:

"Two Per Day" tablets by Life Extension Foundation	1 breakfast, 1 dinner
Simply One multivitamins **"50+ Men"** or **"50+ Women"** by Supernutrition, at Whole Foods	1 per day

—Continued on next page

152

Continued from previous page—

2. **Cysteine**   200 – 600 mg per day
                                                          as food, or in a pill

    Designer Whey protein: 1 rounded scoop at breakfast each day
    provides 200 mg of cysteine. Blend protein into a smoothie with
    some fruit, or mix with some juice and drink.

    or buy pills:
    N-acetylcysteine (NAC) pill, 600 mg   1 per day
                                                          taken anytime

    This is an amino acid that also supports the glutathione
    antioxidant enzyme. It is essentially lung cell repair fuel.

3. **The Probiotic Culturelle**   Take 1 per day
    This product has 10 billion CFU (colony forming units).

4. **Co-Enzyme Q10** pill, 100 mg   Take 1 per day
    This is Natural Killer cell fuel. This part of the "innate" immune
    response greets incoming viruses, then signals the "acquired"
    immune system to get busy.

5. **Know your levels of Vitamin D.**
    In a northern region of the country, many people need 2,000 to
    4,000 international units a day to maintain healthy blood vitamin
    D levels.

6. **L-glutamine powder**   5 grams = 1 rounded teaspoon
                                                          each morning

    Dissolve the powder in 1 oz. of cool water or juice, or just put it
    on your tongue and take a big gulp of water and wash it down.
    This is immune cell fuel, and it boosts glutathione.

Exercise and Immunity

Remember, people with routine physical fitness activity have better immune systems. Their NK cells work better and their IL2 cytokine messaging system is more vigorous.[318] It is not an extreme amount of activity that helps either. In a Japanese study of people age 62 to 79 years old, 10 minutes walking and 10 minutes of leg and arm calisthenics produced important changes in TH1/TH2 balance.[319] The results point toward reducing autoimmune activity, and improving action against the common cold. Exercise also improves the activity of Natural Killer cells and helps vaccines work better.[320]

Auto-immune Disease Concepts

Help for Crohn's Disease, Ulcerative Colitis, Rheumatoid Arthritis, and Other Auto-immune Conditions

This section includes scientific discussions that may be difficult to follow. It is here to open up your awareness to more nutritional possibilities that might benefit you. You should have some individual nutritional counseling to implement the ideas. The drugs used to manage many autoimmune conditions in people are both brilliant and problematic. An increased risk of lymphoma is a huge price to pay for gut or joint comfort. Using sophisticated nutrition plus Chinese energy healing to avert the need for these controversial treatments is worth a try.

There are medical conditions like Crohn's disease, ulcerative colitis, and even multiple sclerosis, that are often labeled autoimmune. People with these diseases go through periods of relatively good health, eperiencing no symptoms. Then they may suddenly experience flare-ups with much discomfort and inflamed tissues. Look back several pages at the TH1 and TH2 response explanation. In essence, a flare-up is a burst of TH2 response activity. Usually there is a burst of IL6 cytokine messaging activity in rheumatoid arthritis,[321] and more of the recently discovered cytokine IL17 in Inflammatory Bowel Disease.[322] Medically it has been generally thought that there are antibodies attacking your own cells in affected body parts, but the picture is more complex, and it is really about immune system dysregulation.

People do have the sense that when they are eating better, their disease stays in remission. In fact, having too much saturated fat and possibly excessive amounts of even good olive oil fat, as well as a deficiency of omega-3 fats, can lead to more unwanted auto-immune disease activity. Foods turn on and off certain immune regulatory genes. The study of nutriton and immune dysregulation has the wonderful name: nutrigenetics.[323]

All in all, this means you could develop a nutrition strategy to reduce autoimmune flare-ups.

- Eat a diet with adequate protein at all three meals, plus eat plenty of fruits and vegetables.

- Support the TH1 response arm of your immune system, to prevent triggering an over active TH2 response. This means being sure the body has adequate amounts of B-complex vitamins, vitamins C and E, plus selenium and zinc.

- Proper glutathione support, with adequate dietary protein, plus some cysteine, L-glutamine or alpha lipoic acid is important too.

- Attend to good gut health. Think about probiotics. Even a dose of friendly yeast can help re-regulate the GI system in Inflammatory Bowel Disease.[324]

It is very important to proceed slowly when starting nutritional support in these autoimmune conditions. Add new elements once every 10 days or so. Rapid immune reconstitution can cause more TH2 activity at first, feeling like a flare-up is happening.

You want good antioxidant foods and basic trace minerals to be the first level of immune system support. You want Natural Killer cells and the TH1 arm of acquired immunity to come into play as a sure and steady process. This way, the TH2 activity fades naturally.

The strategy also includes keeping other systems in their best shape, i.e., no excess inflammation.

Good food and some smart supplements can be very beneficial in autoimmune disease management.

A Few Weight Control Ideas

The Biological Basics

I, like many nutritionists, have sat with hundreds of people who have seriously worked on weight loss for years, often with poor results. Some do achieve a modest reduction in weight. Some get to a trim goal weight. Many hit some weight loss plateau, where despite continued efforts in exercise and in caloric deprivation, they remain stuck. The body just refuses to give up stored fat any more. Then, for all too many people, something happens and the lost pounds return.

Western medicine has come up with no successful food formula for managing weight. When you think about it, over the years, the advice given to people struggling with weight has been all over the map. There were high carb-lower fat diets, then higher fat-lower carb, higher protein, then lower protein diets. The American population is heavier than ever. Scarsdale, South Beach, and Beverly Hills diets have not succeeded where American medicine has failed either. The latest trend is a version of imagined Paleolithic foraging: high fat-high protein-low carbs. Plant-based diets, almost vegan, are also gaining popularity. No plan seems to be a total answer to keeping weight off though.

The difficult part about weight management is that the human metabolic system is built for survival. It knows how to endure famine, starvation or simple caloric restriction. There seems to be something called a "set point", but how to lower it is still a mystery. Fat cells either multiply or swell up to accommodate extra weight, but they never go away with weight loss. It seems that they are unhappy being empty, and lie in ambush, ready to grab any extra calories they can, and swell back up again. They don't wait 'til the end of the day and tally the day's fuel level, and grab the leftovers. Instead, any extra few hundred calories at any meal or snack get whisked off to fat cells right after the food encounter. This is one reason why a work-out program that is continuously pulling stored fat out of fat cells is crucial to maintaining weight loss.

There are still other food elements that are likely at work. If inflammation is not adequately addressed with diet and vitamins, the body tends to accumulate weight. People with more anti-inflammatory omega-3 oils and with more fiber in their diets, maintain lower weights. As mentioned before, hybridized wheat is a suspect in changing metabolism. Dr. Davis' book, *The Wheat Belly Diet*, has been useful for helping many people lose gut-area fat.

We know also, that the gut flora pattern is different in people who struggle with weight. The pattern can start in childhood, and play out over decades. Having lower Bifidobacterium counts and an excess of bacteroides species seems to promote weight gain.[325] Clinical trials providing probiotic supplements to reduce weight are underway with no reliable recommendations yet.

The basic diet detailed throughout this book is still the smartest place to be for managing fat cell inventory. Even more attention to insulin response to meals and snacks will help those who have lost a lot of weight keep it off. Again, I direct your attention to the book, *Always Hungry*, written by David Ludwig MD, PhD in Boston.

Using Exercise as Part of Your Weight Control Plan

Data from the national weight control registry says that people who have maintained a weight loss of 30 lbs or more, for a year or longer, are exercising about 5 hours a week, burning 2,000 calories each week. If you are trying to trim off some unwanted extra weight, make fitness activity the key intervention to reach your goal weight. As people age, under-eating is less productive for weight loss than it was when younger. The body is worried about self-preservation, and metabolic rate will just drop to cope with the starvation it is experiencing.

There are two ways in which your fitness activity can help you lose weight. One is simply yanking fat grams from your muscles, burning them in physical activity. The other is raising metabolic rate through the repair activity that happens after workouts.

As you walk around in your daily routine, your legs are burning a fuel mix that is about 80% starch (glycogen) and 20% fat (triglyceride). If you start walking (or pedalling) faster, and your pulse and breathing rate are up for longer than 20 to 25 minutes, then your muscles think, "Hmmm, I think s/he is traveling over the mountain to trade beads a few villages away; better throw more fat on the fire to get there." So you see in the diagram on the next page, in longer activity sessions, there is an increase of the amount of fat burned in the legs, and a decrease of starch.

Notice that it takes 25 minutes of activity to get to where the switch to more fat-burning happens. Being "in shape" means you are better able to both deliver oyxgen to your muscles and burn fat. In shape is also being able to clear lactic acid and carbon dioxide out of muscles faster. How conditioned you are will alter your fuel mix; more fitness means better ability to burn fat, sparing glycogen reserves. If you are hoping to do fitness activity to pull fat out of your fat cells, then consider one hour walks or bike rides or other cardio sessions, every other day. Your 30-minute activities are good for maintaining muscle health while the 60 to 75=minute sessions are better for emptying fat cells.

For people living at high altitudes, or doing serious cardiovascular exercise, your fuel needs are a little different. Both higher intensity and higher altitude workouts mean lower oxygen levels in muscles. In this situation, muscles burn more glycogen (starch). Keep this in mind if you are on a 3–4 hour hike in higher mountains. You will need more carbohydrate calories per hour.

Exercise science is figuring out that strength training keeps the body busy repairing muscles for an extra day or two after workouts. This burns more calories.[326] You were already trying to do muscle toning activity to reduce

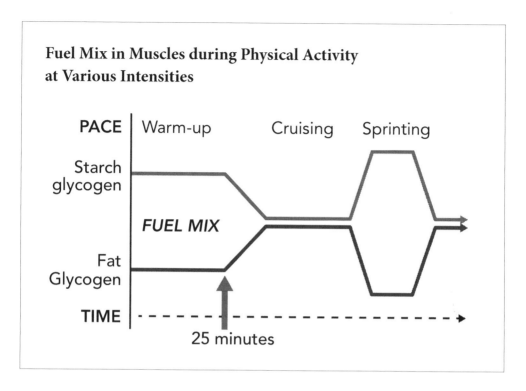

Fuel Mix in Muscles during Physical Activity at Various Intensities

sarcopenia (muscle loss). This added weight-lifting for muscle building is just extra effort on top of that, with weight-loss as a benefit.

How much weight should you lift? You see people at the gym, sweating, and groaning when lifting. This is not necessary for you. There are whole books written on this topic. Chad Waterbury, who writes for Men's Health magazine has a book called *Huge In A Hurry*.[327] Yes, the title sounds like it is a bit more action than you may want. However, in the first 20 pages, Chad describes the principles of resistance exercise that will help you feel smart and confident in your "work out" sessions. He points out that muscles come in small, medium, and large sizes. Gaining strength comes from improving the fitness of the bigger muscles. Too many repeat lifts tires out the small muscles, which won't improve strength, and will mean there is simply more repair work for the body. His system is a breath of fresh air in how it describes gaining strength and fitness without exhausting yourself. His concept is working the big muscles with 6 or 7 reps (repeats of a particular lifting move), and do the reps quickly. Then you're done. Do 2 or 3 sets. Don't struggle to do more, long slow reps; you will just be straining the small muscles. This means more recovery work without much muscle mass gain.

Don't get frustrated if the scale does not reflect weight loss right away for a new, vigorous exercise effort. Distressed muscle may take on more water and this may show up on the scale as an added pound. Sometimes, a pound of added muscle will replace a pound of lost fat, and the scale does not move. Use the improvements in strength and changes in body shape as your measure of progress in weight loss. Trust the process, eventually the weight will come down.

Here is a nice reminder about how food still matters with your exercise program. In a study of people doing strength training, with or without taking 2 grams a day of fish oils, the people with the omega-3 oils showed greater improvements in muscle capacity.[328] You may not have to take 2 more fish oil pills a day to experience these results. Eat your salmon and sardines a few times a week and follow your caveperson plan. All the colors in your fruits and vegetables reduce inflammation, so the body repairs better with that aspect of diet working for you. Remember the whey protein at breakfast helps muscles.[329] You can also take a teaspoon of L-glutamine powder each day to help muscles recuperate. I still encourage you to eat the cave-person food style I have mentioned all along. Portion control does well for weight loss as does attention to caloric density or to glycemic load over the first three months of a weight loss plan at least.[330]

Using Tong Ren Energy Healing
To Boost Nutritional Therapies

In Eastern medicine the flow of Chi, a subtle bioelectrical current, is recognized as a key component of the healing system of the body. Tai Chi, Chigung, and acupuncture get Chi moving. Tong Ren is a new method for doing this.

There are two aspects of Tong Ren to know about. First is that a person can have an acupuncture experience through a brain wave connection with the practitioner. The practitioner taps on an acupuncture teaching figure with a small hammer. This helps the practitioner focus, which generates brain waves. The patient's brain will receive and comprehend the brain wave pattern being generated for them. The patient has an acupuncture treatment experience without being touched or needled. Second, the Tong Ren points that the practitioner touches on the teaching figure correspond to acupuncture points used in Traditional Chinese Medicine. Additionally, some Western medical points are used, like the spinal chord markers used by osteopathic doctors.

Yes, you are wondering, "Can this kind of telepathy actually work?" Well, the answer seems to be a resounding "Yes." We already observe in nature how birds fly in formation, courtesy of some signals from the lead bird. It is not radar, not sonar, not speech; the communication is truly happening even though it is something that we do not yet have the instruments to detect. Similar communication happens with fish and wolves and other creatures.

We can speculate that the mechanism has something to do with quantum physics and quantum entanglement, or the Jungian collective unconscious. Whatever it is, thousands of people including myself are taking advantage of it to help the healing process. I introduce the Tong Ren energy-healing concept here because it offers the chance to generate some remarkable repairs and healings that have no match in Western medicine. For example, I use it to reverse neuropathy (chronic burning and numbness from nerve damage) in people who have had chemotherapy, or who have later stage diabetes. It has also been tremendously helpful to people with multiple sclerosis and Parkinson's disease.

Something about Appreciating Synchronicity

It seems the animal kingdom demonstrates a capacity we can share. The perfectly synchronized movements of birds flying in a flock, or fish swimming in a school are not coordinated by the usual senses of sight, sound, smell, feel or taste, but rather by "brainwave entrainment" with an instinctive commonality. They move in perfect harmony because each is connected with the brainwave energy and patterns of the group.

A natural propensity toward synchronization is even seen in non-biologic systems, such as two pendulum clocks side-by-side on a wall gradually moving into synchronicity. The human brain can change its dominant electroencephalogram patterns toward the frequency of external stimuli.

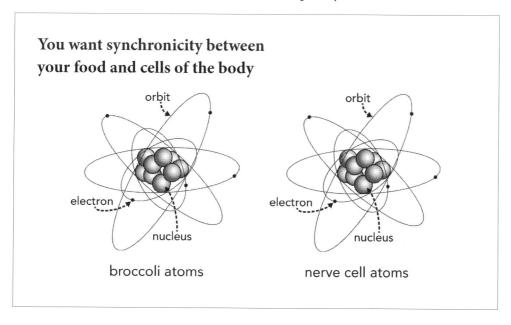

You want synchronicity between your food and cells of the body

broccoli atoms   nerve cell atoms

Several studies have demonstrated a strong tendency for brainwaves of meditating people to synchronize with each other, with no sensory contact. Dr. Carl Jung, Pierre Teilhard de Chardin, Ervin Laszlo, Gary Zukav and others have described the evolving development of a subconscious human connectedness, like a global spirit or brain. As an anthropologist, Teilhard de Chardin traced the natural evolution of life on earth from the development of cells, then plants, through animal and finally human form. This visible biologic evolution then progressed to internal intellectual development, and now finally to globally evolving organization on the level of spirit-energy. We are all part of this upward spiral of energy organization, regardless of our awareness.

In Tong Ren therapy we tap into this vast reserve of healthy bioelectrical patterns and health-sustaining energy. We then use the natural tendency toward synchronicity to bring diseased organs back into harmony with the healthy bioelectric patterns of Tong Ren practitioners, and even more importantly into entrainment with the more powerful global brain. Go to the website http://www.thelivingmatrixmovie.com/free-movie and watch the movie **The Healing Matrix** to get a glimpse into the benefits of energy medicine, and the future it offers everyone. Many people bemoan the lack of scientific rigor in this movie, but I want you to open your mind to the possibilities. The way I see it, "Sometimes you're the Pope and sometimes you're Galileo," when you see radical new ideas.

Here is an additional way to look at Tong Ren energy healing. Modern physics says mass is energy in solid form: $E=MC^2$. We are all made up of atoms, organized into molecules, clumped into constructs like organs and bones. Food is also a collection of atoms and molecules. Remember, atoms have a nucleus containing protons, with electrons spinning around them. The body parts also have orbiting electrons. Let's just imagine that sometimes the energy frequency of various electrons can be slightly out of synchronicity. In this situation, maybe the food and nutrients you eat won't quite be absorbed into some cells as fully as needed. Maybe the electrons of your hormone insulin won't talk to muscle cells as functionally needed.

Eastern medicine practitioners direct the flow of Chi through the body to get all electrons and body parts back into harmony. The benefit may be simply getting all the nutrients of food to fully nourish cells by bringing both food and body energy systems into compatible orbits.

How Tong Ren Energy Healing Happens

People usually experience Tong Ren energy healing in a group setting. Practitioners lead what is called a "healing class." People simply show up at a class; the leader goes around the room and spends a minute or two directing some chi (energy) to each participant. Attendees mention what their health complaints are, generally reporting their doctor's diagnosis. The Tong Ren class leader cannot and does not generate the diagnosis. The leader taps on an acupuncture teaching doll, on the places that correspond to acupuncture points as a way to focus his mind and generate certain brain waves.

The participants simply sit quietly and receive energy. Somehow their nervous systems figure out what energy is coming their way. The energy helps remove blockages in the flow of Chi. Once Chi is moving, the body's own repair systems function better. Class participants generally end up feeling very relaxed and frequently feel some heat or tingling, as their Chi flows. The beauty of Tong Ren energy healing is that it is totally non-invasive: no touching, no needles, no pills.

Tong Ren Healing Points

In tapping the teaching doll, the energy focus may be on blockages as viewed in Western terms, like lumbar nerves L4 and L5 for back pain. It may be a focus at an Eastern energy point, like Conception Vessel 17 for a lung condition such as COPD, lung cancer or emphysema. Energy to Triple Warmer 16 & 17 reduces the side effects of chemotherapy. Energy to Gallbladder 13 reduces anxiety.

People in a class may report a reduction in their back pain, or relief of a headache. Over time, more remarkable improvements happen, such as reversals in Parkinson's and MS symptoms. Many people attend Tong Ren classes when their cancer treatments are not going well.

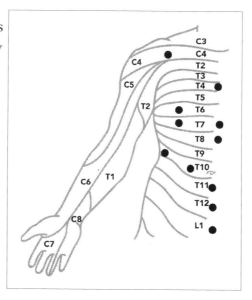

The addition of Chi flow has been a deciding factor in reversing their cancer growth. Researchers like Sarah Know and Timothy Eubank at West Virginia University are studying the role of electrical signals in cancer tumor growth. Michael Levin at Tufts University is connecting cancer gene expression to electrical signaling via the fatty acid butyrate from the microbiome of the colon. This interplay between food, gut flora, cancer genes and bioelectricity is exciting to a nutritionist who adds Chi flow to his nutrition therapies.

Tong Ren is a wonderful accompaniment to nutritional care. I put people on a diabetic diet, and do 7 minutes of Tong Ren energy work with them. They are back in my office in 3 weeks, they are losing weight and their blood sugars are normal and they are feeling better. Sometimes they have gone to a Tong Ren healing class; sometimes they have watched my on-line Youtube treatment videos. I have treated people with residual neuropathy after chemotherapy who use a combination of Coenzyme Q10 and Acetyl L-carnitine and Tong Ren to reverse their nerve pain. It even helps tough conditions like fibromyalgia and chronic fatigue syndrome. I have posted an introductory video that you can watch at www.TongRenNutrition.org. There are a few treatment videos there too.

How to Access some Tong Ren Energy Healing

Go to www.tomtam.com and read testimonials and find out how Tong Ren could be helpful for you. There is also a directory of classes throughout the USA and some other countries. You can also get some healing energy benefits from watching broadcasts live on your computer at www.tongrenstation.com. Click on the "schedule" tab to find a broadcast that works for you.

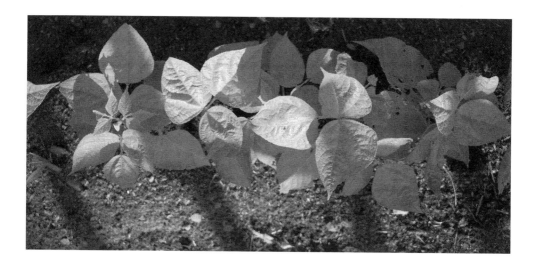

Conclusion _____

In this book are food and nutrition ideas that I learned in thirty years of nutritional counseling. The science of nutrition is still an evolving one. Much of what I offer here could be incomplete in just 5 years. Still, I do think it has much to offer people right now. I hope this book helps sort out conflicting information on what and how to eat. I hope the advice is simple, practical and tasty. And of course, I hope you'll be feeling healthier and more energetic once you are eating as it suggests. I also hope that you may achieve a better state of body repair and you'll move beyond the need for medicines that simply manage symptoms.

Charlie Smigelski, RD

Appendix 1

Supplements I commonly recommend (2018)

Enhanced Multivitamin: 100% RDA for usual vitamins, but also including 100mg magnesium, 100mcg selenium, 5 X RDA for B-complex vitamins, and vitamins C and E.

> Purpose: a nutrient insurance policy for the basics, but also therapeutic for the special needs of people over 50.
>
> Some popular examples:
> - *Two Per Day Tablets* made by Life Extension Foundation
> - *Simply One 50+ Men* or *Simply One 50+ Women* made by SupernutritioN
> - *Active 50+ Once Daily Multivitamin & Mineral* made by Trader Joe's
> - *One Daily Men's 50+* or *One Daily Women's 50+* made by Vitamin Shoppe

Fish Oils: a source of EPA/DHA omega-3 fatty acids

> Purpose: maintain cardiovascular and heart health plus brain cell vitality.
> - A good dose is at least 300mg EPA & 200mg DHA per day.
> - 4 oz salmon or 3.5 oz. sardines provides approx. 1700mg total EPA/DHA.

Evening Primrose Oil: a source of GLA – gamma linolenic acid

> Purpose: fixes dry cracked skin at fingertips, reduces diabetic neuropathy, and raises good HDL cholesterol.
> - Common size pills are 1000mg or 1300 mg; take 2 per day.

L-glutamine amino acid powder

> Purpose: intestine cell repair, immune cell fuel, muscle recovery, glutathione boost.
> - Usual dose, 5 grams (1 teaspoon) a day, taken in a cool liquid

—Continued on next page

Supplements I commonly recommend (2018)

N-acetylcysteine (common abbreviation NAC): a sulfur-containing amino acid

> Purpose: helps lung & liver cells repair, raises HDL cholesterol, boosts glutathione levels.

- Common dose pills are 600mg; take once or twice a day.

Co–enzyme Q10 (Co Q10 for short)**:** an antioxidant, and mitochondria support agent

> Purpose: energy for heart cells, helps lower blood pressure, fuels NK immune cells.

- Common pills are 100mg; take one a day. Take 200mg per day if on a statin drug.

L-carnitine (for muscles and liver) **or Acetyl L-carnitine** (for nerves and brain)

> Purpose: improves fat burning and energy production in the mitochondria.

- 1 gram of L-carnitine a day for a few months helps blood sugar management and helps clean out fatty liver. 500mg a day Acetyl L-carnitine help reverse neuropathies. Best results occur when used along with Co Q10.

Probiotics: supplements that add to the beneficial microbe population in the intestines

> Purpose: probiotics provide repair materials for cells lining the intestine, and make vitamins the body uses. They also support immune cells of the gut.

- I almost always start with the product Culturelle. It is effective and safe, and has been studied in over 125 clinical trials. Buy it at CVS drugstores. JarrodophilusEPS 25 is one I find useful for reducing reflux and lowering cholesterol.

—Continued on next page

Vitamin D3 with vitamin K2: this blend is better than vitamin D3 alone.

> Purpose: prevent vitamin D3 deficiency. The vitamin K2 (menaquinone) helps assure that the extra calcium you absorb goes to bone formation and doesn't clog arteries or land inside joint spaces.

> • Common doses are approximately 2500 units vitamin D3 with 90 micrograms K2. Take 1 a day.

A dose of Chi: I encourage my patients to include some Eastern energy healing treatment with their food and vitamin schemes. For hands on treatment, Tuina massages are hugely effective. Tong Ren therapy is the most accessible surrogate acupuncture. www.TongRenNutrition.org

Appendix 2

Guide to Groceries

The extra–fierce foods are in **bold type**. These are items that have been mentioned in various sections throughout the book.

REPAIR FOODS: **PROTEIN**

Blue fish
Cod
Flounder
Haddock
Herring
Lobster
Salmon
Sardines
Shrimp
Scallops
Trout
Tuna

Whey protein powder
No fat/low-fat cottage
cheese
Egg whites/ EggBeaters
Veggie burger
Turkey breast
Turkey ham
Turkey sausage
Chicken breast
Chicken legs
Chicken thighs
Pork chop

Pork tenderloin
Lite/low-fat cheeses
Omega-3 eggs

Grass-fed is best:
Lamb chops
Lean beef
Cheese, especially
    goat & sheep

Collagen peptides

CALCIUM FOODS

Almond milk
Low fat/skim milk

Dark greens
Yogurt

Bone Repair
Algae sources
www.Algaecal.com

ANTIOXIDANT & IMMUNE SYSTEM FOODS: **VEGETABLES**

Asparagus
Bok choy
Broccoli
Brussels sprouts
Cabbage
Carrots
Cauliflower
Celery
Collard greens
Cucumbers
Dandelion greens

Dark green lettuce
Eggplant
Green/yellow beans
Green/red/hot peppers
Kale
Mushrooms
Mustard greens
Okra
Onions
Parsley
Parsnips

Pea pods
Purslane
Spinach
Summer squash
Swiss chard
Tomatoes
Tomato sauce
Winter squash
Zucchini squash

—Continued on next page

Guide to Groceries

ANTIOXIDANT & IMMUNE SYSTEM FOODS: **FRUITS**

It's better to eat solid fruit than drink juices.

Apples
Applesauce
Apricots
Bananas
Blackberries
Blueberries
Cantaloupe
Clementines
Grapefruit
Honeydew
Kiwis
Lychee
Mangos
Nectarines
Oranges

Papaya
Peaches
Pears
Pineapple
Plums
Pomegranate
Raspberries
Red grapes
Strawberries
Watermelon

Dried fruit (extra sweet)
Dates
Figs
Raisins
Cran-raisins

4 oz juices
Apricot nectar
Grape juice
Grapefruit juice
Orange juice
Pineapple juice
Red pomegranate
   juice

ENERGY FOODS: **STARCHES & CARBOHYDRATES**

Black beans
Black-eyed peas
Chickpeas
Hummus
Lentils
Lima beans
Navy beans
Pinto beans
Red kidney beans
Sweet potatoes
White kidney beans
Yams

100% Rye bread

Barley
Buckwheat
Cheerios
Corn
Corn tortillas
Millet
Oat Bran
Oatmeal
Peas
Plantain
Potatoes
Quinoa
Rice

Careful
Bagels
Cakes
Candy
Cookies
Muffins
Noodles
Pancakes
Saltines
Spaghetti
Waffles
White bread
Whole wheat bread

—Continued on next page

ENERGY FOODS: **FATS & OILS**

Almonds	**Chia seeds**	*Be modest*
Brazil nuts	**Ground flax seeds**	Butter (grass fed is
Cashews	Hemp seeds	nice)
Hazelnuts	Pepitas	Lard
Macadamia nuts	Pumpkin seeds	
Peanuts	Sesame seeds	*Avoid*
Pecans	Sunflower seeds	Canola oil
Pine nuts		Corn oil
Pistachio nuts	Avocado	Cotton seed oil
Soy nuts	Coconut oil	Cream cheese
Walnuts	**Olives**	Fried fast foods
	Olive oil	Safflower oil
	Peanut oil	Stick margarine
		Vegetable oil

Using The Guide To Groceries

The Protein Columns

Eat protein at breakfast as well as at lunch and supper. Fish in bold type contain omega-3's, which are super good for you. Yes, they are brain food, and prevent heart attacks. Seafood is fine, but have it cooked, not raw. Shrimp and lobster don't contain a lot of cholesterol. Research has figured out that they have useful many sterols that actually lower cholesterol. Some tuna has too much mercury; careful. Chicken and turkey are ok too; they have little fat. Lean pork is fine too; it is the other white meat these days. Moving to beef, just keep to the lean items, like a sirloin steak; grass fed would be extra good. Dairy fat is bad news for people worried about cholesterol; low fat dairy products are ok though. Eggs are totally fine. Buy omega-3 eggs if you can; the chickens were fed better. Milk and yogurt come low fat; they are just a 1/2 size portion of protein. They have about 8 or 10 grams of protein per serving, and you are usually looking for 20 to 30 grams at a meal. Add a scoop of Designer whey protein powder to make the milk in your cereal be a full protein serving.

The Vegetable Columns

All vegetables are great. The ones in bold type are seriously nutritious. They have more carotenes, or more potassium, or both, plus other minerals. Eat tons at lunch too.

The Fruit Columns

All fruits are good. The ones in bold type deserve more of your attention. They have more vitamin C, or more potassium, or both. Eat fruit 3 or 4 times a day

The Starch Columns

Eating more foods from the first column is a brilliant idea. Notice that beans are really a starch. Eighty percent of their calories come from carbohydrate, and just 20% from protein. Then eat yams, peas , corn, and plantain. Next, eat whole grains. Rye is <u>much</u> better than wheat. The foods in the column cause the slowest blood sugar rise. The foods in the last column have the least vitamins and minerals, plus added fat and sugar.

The Oils Columns

A handful of nuts and one of seeds each day is good for your health. As much as possible, have the oil that goes into your body be more from foods like nuts and seeds, plus from fish. Cook with olive, coconut, and peanut oils, but use them in just modest amounts. Notice that canola oil, corn oil, safflower oil, and vegetable oil are trouble; they are somewhat inflammatory. Enjoy butter in modest amounts with special foods. Buy grass-fed butter when you can.

As you assemble meals, think about having some repair foods (protein), some immune support foods (vegetables or fruit) and then some energy foods (a starch and a fat mix).

Even with all these great foods, take an antioxidant multivitamin for best health.

Reference Notes

[1]   http://changingminds.org/explanations/needs/maslow.htm

[2]   O'Keefe JH Jr, Cordain L. Cardiovascular disease resulting from a diet and lifestyle at odds with our Paleolithic genome: how to become a 21st-century hunter-gatherer. Mayo Clin Proc. 2004;79(1):101-8.

[3]   Gaffney-Stomberg E, Insogna KL, Rodriguez NR, Kerstetter JE. Increasing dietary protein requirements in elderly people for optimal muscle and bone health. J Am Geriatr Soc. 2009;57(6):1073-9.

[4]   Willett W. Fruits, Vegetables, and Cancer Prevention: Turmoil in the Produce Section. J Natl Cancer Inst 102(8): 510-11. **9 a day for cancer more veggies than you think**

[5]   Sponheimer M, Lee-Thorp JA. Isotopic evidence for the diet of an early hominid, Australopithecus africanus. Science. 1999;283(5400):368-70.

[6]   Wolever TM, Mehling C. Long-term effect of varying the source or amount of dietary carbohydrate on postprandial plasma glucose, insulin, triacylglycerol, and free fatty acid concentrations in subjects with impaired glucose tolerance. Am J Clin Nutr. 2003;77(3):612-21.

[7]   Frank R, Berndt ER, Donohue J, Epstein A, Rosenthal M. Trends in Direct-to-Consumer Advertising of Prescription Drugs. Kaiser Family Foundation Document. 2002.

[8]   Iannuzzi-Sucich M, Prestwood KM, Kenny AM. Prevalence of sarcopenia and predictors of skeletal muscle mass in healthy, older men and women. J Gerontol A Biol Sci Med Sci. 2002;57(12):M772-7.

[9]   Simopoulos AP, Visioli F. More on Mediterranean Diets. World Review of Nutrition and Dietetics, Vol 97: P 68. Karger 2007

[10] Simopoulos AP, Visioli F. More on Mediterranean Diets. World Review of Nutrition and Dietetics, Vol 97: P 73. Karger 2007.

[11] David Heber, MD PhD. What Color Is Your Diet? Regan Books/Harper Collins, 2001.

[12] Kimm SY, Glynn NW, Aston CE, Damcott CM, Poehlman ET, Daniels SR, Ferrell RE Racial differences in the relation between uncoupling protein genes and resting energy expenditure. Am J Clin Nutr. 2002;75(4):714-9.

[13] Hurst S, Rees SG, Randerson PF, Caterson B, Harwood JL. Contrasting effects of n-3 and n-6 fatty acids on cyclooxygenase-2 in model systems for arthritis. Lipids. 2009;44(10):889-96.

[14] Min Y, Lowy C, Islam S, Khan FS, Swaminathan R. Relationship between red cell membrane fatty acids and adipokines in individuals with varying insulin sensitivity. Eur J Clin Nutr. 2011 Jun;65(6):690-5. Epub 2011 Mar 9.

[15] Smith WL. Cyclooxygenases, peroxide tone and the allure of fish oil. Curr Opin Cell Biol. 2005 Apr;17(2):174-82.

[16] Merino DM, Ma DW, Mutch DM. Genetic variation in lipid desaturases and its impact on the development of human disease. Lipids Health Dis. 2010. 18;9:63.

[17] Schubert R, Kitz R, Beermann C, Rose MA, Lieb A, Sommerer PC, Moskovits J, Alberternst H, Böhles HJ, Schulze J, Zielen S. Effect of n-3 polyunsaturated fatty acids in asthma after low-dose allergen challenge. Int Arch Allergy Immunol. 2009;148(4):321-

[18] Tapiero H, Ba GN, Couvreur P, Tew KD. Polyunsaturated fatty acids (PUFA) and eicosanoids in human health and pathologies. Biomed Pharmacother. 2002 Jul;56(5):215-22.

[19] Stoll AL, Locke CA, Marangell LB, Severus WE. Omega-3 fatty acids and bipolar disorder: a review. Prostaglandins Leukot Essent Fatty Acids. 1999;60(5-6):329-37.

[20] Johnson EJ, Schaeffer EL. Potential role of dietary n-3 fatty acids in the prevention of dementia and macular degeneration. Am J Clin Nutr. 2006;83(6 Suppl):1494S-1498S..

[21] Frisardi V, Panza F, Seripa D, Imbimbo BP, Vendemiale G, Pilotto A, Solfrizzi V. Nutraceutical properties of Mediterranean diet and cognitive decline: possible underlying mechanisms. J Alzheimers Dis. 2010;22(3):715-40.

[22] Conquer JA, Holub BJ. Supplementation with an algae source of docosahexaenoic acid increases (n-3) fatty acid status and alters selected risk factors for heart disease in vegetarian subjects. J Nutr. 1996;126(12):3032-9.

[23] http://www.amazon.com/s/?ie=UTF8&keywords=dha+gummy&tag=googhydr-20&index=aps&hvadid=12499647107&ref=pd_sl_4kwisxtzfu_b

[24] Hibbeln JR, Nieminen LR, Blasbalg TL, Riggs JA, Lands WE. Healthy intakes of n-3 and n-6 fatty acids: estimations considering worldwide diversity. Am J Clin Nutr. 2006;83(6 Suppl):1483S-1493S.

[25] Gesch CB, Hammond SM, Hampson SE, Eves A, Crowder MJ. Influence of supplementary vitamins, minerals and essential fatty acids on the antisocial behaviour of young adult prisoners. Randomised, placebo-controlled trial. Br J Psychiatry. 2002;181:22-8.

[26] Freeman MP, Hibbeln JR, Wisner KL, Davis JM, Mischoulon D, Peet M, Keck PE Jr, Marangell LB, Richardson AJ, Lake J, Stoll AL. Omega-3 fatty acids: evidence basis for treatment and future research in psychiatry. J Clin Psychiatry. 2006;67(12):1954-67.

[27] National Center for Health Statistics. Mortality Report. Hyattsville, MD: U.S. Department of Health and Human Services; 2002.

[28] US Department of Health and Human Services, National Center for Health Statistics. Health, United States, 2010: With Special Feature on Death and Dying. Hyattsville, MD. 2011. Table 94: Prescription Drug Use In The Last Month, page 318, Trend Tables.

[29] Downs JR, Clearfield M, Weis S, Whitney E, Shapiro DR, Beere PA, Langendorfer A, Stein EA, Kruyer W, Gotto AM Jr.Primary prevention of acute coronary events with lovastatin in men and women with average cholesterol levels: results of AFCAPS/

TexCAPS. Air Force/Texas Coronary Atherosclerosis Prevention Study. JAMA. 1998;279(20):1615-22.

[30] Bengmark S. Advanced glycation and lipoxidation end products--amplifiers of inflammation: the role of food. JPEN J Parenter Enteral Nutr. 2007;31(5):430-40.

[31] Gil A, Bengmark S. [Advanced glycation and lipoxidation end products--amplifiers of inflammation: the role of food]. Nutr Hosp. 2007;22(6):625-40.

[32] William Evans, PhD & Irving Rosenberg, MD, Biomarkers. Fireside, 1992.

[33] Campbell WW, Trappe TA, Wolfe RR, Evans WJ. The recommended dietary allowance for protein may not be adequate for older people to maintain skeletal muscle. J Gerontol A Biol Sci Med Sci. 2001;56(6):M373-80.

[34] Marco V. Narici†* and Nicola Maffulli. Sarcopenia: characteristics, mechanisms and functional significance. British Medical Bulletin 2010; 95: 139–159

[35] Douglas Paddon-Jones and Blake B. Rasmussen. Dietary protein recommendations and the prevention of sarcopenia: Protein, amino acid metabolism and therapy. Curr Opin Clin Nutr Metab Care. 2009; 12(1): 86–90.

[36] Iglay HB, Apolzan JW, Gerrard DE, Eash JK, Anderson JC, Campbell WW. Moderately increased protein intake predominately from egg sources does not influence whole body, regional, or muscle composition responses to resistance training in older people. J Nutr Health Aging. 2009;13(2):108-14.

[37] Albert CM, Hennekens CH, O'Donnell CJ, Ajani UA, Carey VJ, Willett WC, Ruskin JN, Manson JE. Fish consumption and risk of sudden cardiac death. JAMA. 1998 ;279(1):23-8.

[38] O'Keefe JH Jr, Cordain L. Cardiovascular disease resulting from a diet and lifestyle at odds with our Paleolithic genome: how to become a 21st-century hunter-gatherer. Mayo Clin Proc. 2004;79(1):101-8.

[39] Donald R. Davis, PhD, FACN, Melvin D. Epp, PhD and Hugh D. Riordan, MD Changes in USDA Food Composition Data for 43 Garden Crops, 1950 to 1999 Journal of the American College of Nutrition, 2004. 23:(6): 669–682.

[40] United Kingdom, Medical Research Council, Ministry of Agriculture .... Royal Society of Chemistry; http://www.mineralresourcesint.co.uk/pdf/mineral_deplet.pdf

[41] Velandia B, Centor RM, McConnell V, Shah M. Scurvy is still present in developed countries. J Gen Intern Med. 2008;23(8):1281-4.

[42] Hibbeln JR. From homicide to happiness--a commentary on omega-3 fatty acids in human society. Cleave Award Lecture. Nutr Health. 2007;19(1-2):9-19.

[43] Selhub J, Jacques PF, Bostom AG, D'Agostino RB, Wilson PW, Belanger AJ, O'Leary DH, Wolf PA, Schaefer EJ, Rosenberg IH. Association between plasma homocysteine concentrations and extracranial carotid-artery stenosis. N Engl J Med. 1995;332(5):286-91.

[44] Johansson M, Relton C, Ueland PM, et al. Serum B vitamin levels and risk of lung cancer. JAMA. 2010 Jun;303(23):2377-85.

45   Altura BM, Altura BT. Magnesium and cardiovascular biology: an important link between cardiovascular risk factors and atherogenesis. Cell Mol Biol Res. 1995;41(5):347-59.

46   Durlach J, Bac P, Durlach V, Rayssiguier Y, Bara M, Guiet-Bara A. Magnesium status and ageing: an update. Magnes Res. 1998;11(1):25-42.

47   Rylander R, Mégevand Y, Lasserre B, Amstutz W, Granbom S. Moderate alcohol consumption and urinary excretion of magnesium and calcium. Scand J Clin Lab Invest. 2001;61(5):401-5.

48   Holick MF. Calcium and Vitamin D. Diagnostics and Therapeutics. Clin Lab Med. 2000 Sep;20(3):569-90.

49   Lips P, Bouillon R, et al. Reducing fracture risk with calcium and vitamin D. Clin Endocrinol (Oxf) 2010; 73(3):277-85.

50   Dawson-Hughes B. Serum 25-hydroxyvitamin D and muscle atrophy in the elderly. Proc Nutr Soc. 2011. ___ epub so far

51   Khokhar JS, Brett AS, Desai A. Vitamin D deficiency masquerading as metastatic cancer: a case series. Am J Med Sci. 2009;337(4):245-7.

52   Kampman MT, Steffensen LH. The role of vitamin D in multiple sclerosis. J Photochem Photobiol B. 2010;101(2):137-41.

53   Porojnicu AC, Robsahm TE, Dahlback A, Berg JP, Christiani D, Bruland OS, Moan J. Seasonal and geographical variations in lung cancer prognosis in Norway. Does Vitamin D from the sun play a role? Lung Cancer. 2007;55(3):263-70.

54   Holick MF. Vitamin D and sunlight: strategies for cancer prevention and other health benefits. Clin J Am Soc Nephrol. 2008;3(5):1548-54.

55   Simonsen L, Taylor RJ, Viboud C, Miller MA, Jackson LA. Mortality benefits of influenza vaccination in elderly people: an ongoing controversy. Lancet Infect Dis. 2007;7(10):658-66.

56   Cannell JJ, Vieth R, Umhau JC, Holick MF, Grant WB, Madronich S, Garland CF, Giovannucci E. Epidemic influenza and vitamin D. Epidemiol Infect. 2006;134(6):1129-40.

57   Berry DJ, Hesketh K, Power C, Hyppönen E. Vitamin D status has a linear association with seasonal infections and lung function in British adults. Br J Nutr. 2011;106(9):1433-40.

58   Cannell JJ, Zasloff M, Garland CF, Scragg R, Giovannucci E. On the epidemiology of influenza. Virol J. 2008;5:29.

59   Aloia JF, Li-Ng. Correspondence, Re: Epidemic Influenza and Vitamin D. Epidemiol Infect. 2007; 135(7): 1095–1098.

60   Urashima M, Segawa T, et al. Randomized trial of vitamin D supplementation to prevent seasonal influenza A in schoolchildren. Am J Clin Nutr. 2010 91(5): 1255-60.

[61] Wouters-Wesseling W, Rozendaal M, Snijder M, Graus Y, Rimmelzwaan G, De Groot L, Bindels J. Effect of a complete nutritional supplement on antibody response to influenza vaccine in elderly people. J Gerontol A Biol Sci Med Sci. 2002;57(9):M563-6.

[62] Meydani SN, Meydani M, Blumberg JB, Leka LS, Siber G, Loszewski R, Thompson C, Pedrosa MC, Diamond RD, Stollar BD. Vitamin E supplementation and in vivo immune response in healthy elderly subjects. A randomized controlled trial. JAMA. 1997;277(17):1380-6.

[63] Glueck CJ1, Jetty V1, Rothschild M1, et al. Associations between Serum 25-hydroxyvitamin D and Lipids, Lipoprotein Cholesterols, and Homocysteine. N Am J Med Sci. 2016;8(7):284-90.

[64] Fraternale A, Paoletti MF, Casabianca A, Oiry J, Clayette P, Vogel JU, Cinatl J Jr, et al. Antiviral and immunomodulatory properties of new pro-glutathione (GSH) molecules. Curr Med Chem. 2006;13(15):1749-55.

[65] Stey C, Steurer J, Bachmann S, Medici TC, Tramèr MR. The effect of oral N-acetylcysteine in chronic bronchitis: a quantitative systematic review. Eur Respir J. 2000;16(2):253-62.

[66] Decramer M, Rutten-van Mölken M, Dekhuijzen PN, Troosters T, van Herwaarden C, Pellegrino R, van Schayck CP, Olivieri D, Del Donno M, De Backer W, Lankhorst I, Ardia A. Effects of N-acetylcysteine on outcomes in chronic obstructive pulmonary disease (Bronchitis Randomized on NAC Cost-Utility Study, BRONCUS): a randomised placebo-controlled trial. Lancet. 2005;365(9470):1552-60.

[67] Weatherall M, Clay J, James K, Perrin K, Shirtcliffe P, Beasley R. Dose-response relationship of inhaled corticosteroids and cataracts: a systematic review and meta-analysis. Respirology. 2009;14(7):983-90.

[68] Julius M, Lang C, Gleiberman L, Harbijrg E, et al. Glutathione and morbidity in a community-based sample of elderly. ClinEpidemiol 1994. 47: (9,)1021-1026.

[69] Bengmark S. Econutrition and health maintenance: A new concept to prevent inflammation, ulceration and sepsis. Clin Nutr 1996;15:1–10.

[70] Andrew Weil, MD Spontaneous Healing, Balantine Books, 1995, pp156-9.

[71] Castro-Giner F, Künzli N, Jacquemin B, Forsberg B, de Cid R, Sunyer J, Jarvis D, Briggs D, Vienneau D, Norback D, González JR, Guerra S, Janson C, Antó JM, Wjst M, Heinrich J, Estivill X, Kogevinas M. Traffic-related air pollution, oxidative stress genes, and asthma (ECHRS). Environ Health Perspect. 2009;117(12):1919-24.

[72] Wood LG, Gibson PG. Reduced circulating antioxidant defenses are associated with airway hyper-responsiveness, poor control and severe disease pattern in asthma. Br J Nutr. 2010 Mar;103(5):735-41.

[73] Produce For Better Health Foundation; The State of America's Plate 2005: study on America's Consumption of Fruit and Vegetable. AC Neilsen, 2004 survey. PBH Foundation, 7465 Lancaster Pike Suite J, 2nd Floor, Hockessin, DE 19707

[74] Simopoulos AP. Evolutionary aspects of omega-3 fatty acids in the food supply. Prostaglandins Leukot Essent Fatty Acids. 1999; 60(5-6): 421-9.

176

75 Stampfer MJ, Hennekens CH, Manson JE, Colditz GA, Rosner B, Willett WC. Vitamin E consumption and the risk of coronary disease in women. N Engl J Med. 1993;328(20):1444-9.

76 Pfister R, Sharp SJ, Luben R, Wareham NJ, Khaw KT. Plasma vitamin C predicts incident heart failure in men and women in European Prospective Investigation into Cancer and Nutrition-Norfolk prospective study. Am Heart J. 2011;162(2):246-5

77 Gurven M, Kaplan H, Winking J, Eid Rodriguez D, Vasunilashorn S, Kim JK, Finch C, Crimmins E. Inflammation and infection do not promote arterial aging and cardiovascular disease risk factors among lean horticulturalists. PLoS One. 2009;4(8):e6590.

78 www westonprice org

79 DrogeW. Oxidative stress and ageing: is ageing a cysteine deficiency syndrome? Philos Trans R Soc Lond B Biol Sci. 2005;360(1464):2355-72.

80 Briefel RR, Bialostosky K, Kennedy-Stephenson J, McDowell MA, Ervin RB, Wright JD. Zinc intake of the U.S. population: findings from the third National Health and Nutrition Examination Survey, 1988-1994. J Nutr. 2000;130(5S Suppl):1367S-73S.

81 Tamblyn R, Equale T, Winslade , Doran P . The incidence and determinants of primary nonadherence with prescribed medication in primary care: a cohort study. Ann Intern Med. 2014;160(7):441-50.

82 Bourre JM. Effects of nutrients (in food) on the structure and function of the nervous system: update on dietary requirements for brain. Part 1: micronutrients. J Nutr Health Aging. 2006:377-85.

83 Schaefer EJ, Bongard V, Beiser AS, Lamon-Fava S, Robins SJ, Au R, Tucker KL, Kyle DJ, Wilson PW, Wolf PA. Plasma phosphatidylcholine docosahexaenoic acid content and risk of dementia and Alzheimer disease: the Framingham Heart Study. Arch Neurol. 2006;63(11):1545-50.

84 Hibbeln JR, Nieminen LR, Blasbalg TL, Riggs JA, Lands WE. Healthy intakes of n-3 and n-6 fatty acids: estimations considering worldwide diversity. Am J Clin Nutr. 2006 Jun (6 Suppl):1483S-1493S.

85 Circulation. 2002; 106: 2747-57.

AHA Scientific Statement
Fish Consumption, Fish Oil, Omega-3 Fatty Acids, and Cardiovascular Disease
TABLE 5. Summary of Recommendations for Omega-3 Fatty Acid Intake

Population	Recommendation
Patients without documented CHD	Eat a variety of (preferably oily) fish at least twice a week Includes oils and foods rich in alpha-linolenic acid (flaxseed, camola, and soybean oils; flaxseed and walnuts

Population	Recommendation
Patients with documented CHD	Consume approximately 1 g of EPA+DHA per day, preferably from oily fish. EPA+DHA supplements could be considered in consultation with the physician.
Patients needing triglyceride lowering	Two to four grams of EPA+DHA per day provided as capsules under a physician's care

[86] Dietary supplementation with n-3 polyunsaturated fatty acids and vitamin E after myocardial infarction: results of the GISSI-Prevenzione trial. Gruppo Italiano per lo Studio della Sopravvivenza nell'Infarto miocardico. Lancet. 1999;354(9177):447-55.

[87] Gerster H. Can adults adequately convert alpha-linolenic acid (18:3n-3) to eicosapentaenoic acid (20:5n-3) and docosahexaenoic acid (22:6n-3)? Int J Vitam Nutr Res. 1998;68(3):159-73.

[88] Johnson EJ, Schaefer EJ. Potential role of dietary n-3 fatty acids in the prevention of dementia and macular degeneration. Am J Clin Nutr. 2006;83(6 Suppl):1494S-1498S.

[89] Calabrese V, Cornelius C, Mancuso C, Lentile R, Stella AM, Butterfield DA. Redox homeostasis and cellular stress response in aging and neurodegeneration. Methods Mol Biol. 2010;610:285-308.

[90] Debette S, Beiser A, Hoffmann U, Decarli C, O'Donnell CJ, Massaro JM, Au R, Himali JJ, Wolf PA, Fox CS, Seshadri S. Visceral fat is associated with lower brain volume in healthy middle-aged adults. Ann Neurol. 2010;68(2):136-44.

[91] Scarmeas N, Luchsinger JA, Schupf N, Brickman AM, Cosentino S, Tang MX, Stern Y. Physical Activity, Diet, and Risk of Alzheimer Disease. JAMA 2009; 302(6): 627-37.

[92] Tan ZS, Beiser AS, Fox CS, Au R, Himali JJ, Debette S, Decarli C, Vasan RS, Wolf PA, Seshadri S. Association of metabolic dysregulation with volumetric brain magnetic resonance imaging and cognitive markers of subclinical brain aging in middle-aged adults: the Framingham Offspring Study. Diabetes Care. 2011;34(8):1766-70.

[93] Kawahara M, Kuroda Y. Molecular mechanism of neurodegeneration induced by Alzheimer's beta-amyloid protein: channel formation and disruption of calcium homeostasis. Brain Res Bull. 2000;53(4):389-97.

[94] Kawahara M, Kuroda Y. Intracellular calcium changes in neuronal cells induced by Alzheimer's beta-amyloid protein are blocked by estradiol and cholesterol. Cell Mol Neurobiol. 2001;21(1):1-13.

[95] Potempa LA, Kubak BM, Gewurz H. Effect of divalent metal ions and pH upon the binding reactivity of human serum amyloid P component, a C-reactive protein homologue, for zymosan. Preferential reactivity in the presence of copper and acidic pH. J Biol Chem. 1985;260(22):12142-7.

[96] Krikorian R, Shidler MD, Nash TA, Kalt W, Vinqvist-Tymchuk MR, Shukitt-Hale B, Joseph JA. Blueberry supplementation improves memory in older adults. J Agric Food Chem. 2010;58(7):3996-4000.

[97] Joseph JA, Shukitt-Hale B, Willis LM. Grape juice, berries, and walnuts affect brain aging and behavior. J Nutr. 2009;139(9):1813S-7S.

98 Rayssiguier Y, Durlach J, Gueux E, Rock E, Mazur A. Magnesium and ageing. I. Experimental data: importance of oxidative damage. Magnes Res. 1993;6(4):369-78.

99 Wallwork JC. Zinc and the central nervous system. Prog Food Nutr Sci. 1987;11(2):203-47.

100 Naurath HJ, Joosten E, Riezler R, Stabler SP, Allen RH, Lindenbaum J. Effects of vitamin B12, folate, and vitamin B6 supplements in elderly people with normal serum vitamin concentrations. Lancet. 1995;346(8967):85-9.

101 McCaddon A, Hudson P, Ellis D, Hill D, Lloyd A. Correspondance. Lancet 2002; 360 (9327):173

102 Smith AD, Smith SM, de Jager CA, Whitbread P, Johnston C, Agacinski G, Oulhaj A, Bradley KM, Jacoby R, Refsum H. Homocysteine-lowering by B vitamins slows the rate of accelerated brain atrophy in mild cognitive impairment: a randomized controlled trial. PLoS One. 2010;5(9):e12244.

103 Marcuard SP, Albernaz L, Khazanie PG. Omeprazole therapy causes malabsorption of cyanocobalamin (vitamin B12) Ann Intern Med. 1994;120(3):211-5.

104 Bains J, Birks JS, Dening TR. The efficacy of antidepressants in the treatment of depression in dementia. Cochrane Database Syst Rev. 2002;(4):CD003944.

105 Möller HJ. [Relativising the significance of the results of metaanalyses: comments on the metaanalysis by Kirsch et al. 2008 regarding the effectiveness of modern antidepressants]. MMW Fortschr Med. 2009;151(13):80-3.

106 Das UN. Folic acid and polyunsaturated fatty acids improve cognitive function and prevent depression, dementia, and Alzheimer's disease--but how and why? Prostaglandins Leukot Essent Fatty Acids. 2008;78(1):11-9.

107 Catena-Dell'Osso M, Bellantuono C, Consoli G, Baroni S, Rotella F, Marazziti D. Inflammatory and neurodegenerative pathways in depression: a new avenue for antidepressant development? Curr Med Chem. 2011;18(2):245-55.

108 Maes M, Yirmyia R, Noraberg J, Brene S, Hibbeln J, Perini G, Kubera M, Bob P, Lerer B, Maj M. The inflammatory & neurodegenerative (I&ND) hypothesis of depression: leads for future research and new drug developments in depression. Metab Brain Dis. 2009;24(1):27-53.

109 The Sharp Brains Guide to Brain Fitness: 18 Interviews with Scientists, Practical Advice, and Product Reviews, To Keep Your Brain Sharp. Alvaro Fernandez & Elkhonon Goldberg.

110 Relaxation Revolution: Enhancing Your Personal Health Through the Science and Genetics of Mind Body Healing. Benson

111 Richard A. Kronmal, PhD; Kevin C. Cain, PhD; Zhan Ye, MD; Gilbert S. Omenn, MD, PhD. Total Serum Cholesterol Levels and Mortality Risk as a Function of Age A Report Based on the Framingham Data. Arch Intern Med. 1993;153(9):1065-1073.

112 Krumholz HM, Seeman TE, Merrill SS, et al. Lack of association between cholesterol and coronary heart disease mortality and morbidity and all-cause mortality in persons older than 70 years. JAMA. 1994;272(17):1335-40.

[113] Schatz IJ, Masaki K, Yano K, Chen R, Rodriguez BL, Curb JD. Cholesterol and all-cause mortality in elderly people from the Honolulu Heart Program: a cohort study. Lancet. 2001 Aug 4;358(9279):351-5

[114] Capurso A. Lipid metabolism and cardiovascular risk: should hypercholesterolemia be treated in the elderly? J Hypertens Suppl. 1992;10(2):S65-8.

[115] Nago N, Ishikawa S, Goto T, Kayaba K. Low cholesterol is associated with mortality from stroke, heart disease, and cancer: the Jichi Medical School Cohort Study. J Epidemiol. 2011;21(1):67-74.

[116] Leibowitz M, Karpati T, Cohen-Stavi CJ. Association Between Achieved Low-Density Lipoprotein Levels and Major Adverse Cardiac Events in Patients With Stable Ischemic Heart Disease Taking Statin Treatment. JAMA Intern Med. 2016;176(8):1105-13.

[117] Sakatani T1, Shirayama T, Suzaki Y, et al. The association between cholesterol and mortality in heart failure. Comparison between patients with and without coronary artery disease. Int Heart J. 2005;46(4):619-29.

[118] Therapeutics Initiative: Therapeutics Letter #77. Do statins have a role in primary prevention? An update. October 18, 2010.

[119] Find link to the letter at: http://www.cas.usf.edu/news/s/176.

[120] Mozaffarian D. Effects of dietary fats versus carbohydrates on coronary heart disease: a review of the evidence. Curr Atheroscler Rep. 2005;7(6):435-45.

[121] Mozaffarian D. The great fat debate: taking the focus off of saturated fat. J Am Diet Assoc. 2011 May;111(5):665-6.

[122] http://mycourses.med.harvard.edu/MediaPlayer/Player.aspx?v={FD6EDE1D-759F-4D31-A162-E3767C12155B}

[123] Mediterranean diet, traditional risk factors, and the rate of cardiovascular complications after myocardial infarction: final report of the Lyon Diet Heart Study. Circulation 1999; 99(6): 779-85.

[124] Joshipura KJ, Hu FB, Manson JE, Stampfer MJ, Rimm EB, Speizer FE, Colditz G, Ascherio A, Rosner B, Spiegelman D, Willett WC. The Effect of Fruit and Vegetable Intake on Risk for Coronary Heart Disease. Ann Intern Med. 2001;134:1106-1114.

[125] Kannel WB. Cholesterol and risk of coronary heart disease and mortality in men. Clin Chem. 1988;34(8B):B53-9.

[126] Abramson, John. Overdosed America, The Broken Promise of American Medicine.

[127] Sugiyama T, Tsugawa Y, Tseng CH, Kobayashi Y, Shapiro MF. Different time trends of caloric and fat intake between statin users and nonusers among US adults: gluttony in the time of statins? JAMA Intern Med 2014 Jul;174(7):1038-45.

[128] Li JZ, Chen ML, Wang S, Dong J, Zeng P, Hou LW. Apparent protective effect of high density lipoprotein against coronary heart disease in the elderly. Chin Med J (Engl). 2004;117(4):511-5.

[129] Kinscherf R, Cafaltzis K, Röder F, Hildebrandt W, Edler L, Deigner HP, Breitkreutz R, Feussner G, Kreuzer J, Werle E, Michel G, Metz J, Dröge W. Cholesterol levels linked to abnormal plasma thiol concentrations and thiol/disulfide redox status in hyperlipidemic subjects. Free Radic Biol Med. 2003;35(10):1286-92.

[130] Franceschini G, Werba JP, Safa O, Gikalov I, Sirtori CR. Dose-related increase of HDL-cholesterol levels after N-acetylcysteine in man. Pharmacol Res. 1993;28(3):213-8.

[131] Miller TL, Wolin MJ. Pathways of Acetate, Propionate, and Butyrate Formation by the Human Fecal Microbial Flora. Applied and Environmental Microbiology; 62(5):1589–1592.

[132] Kallio P, Kolehmainen M, Laaksonen DE, Kekäläinen J, Salopuro T, Sivenius K, Pulkkinen L, Mykkänen HM, Niskanen L, Uusitupa M, Poutanen KS. Dietary carbohydrate modification induces alterations in gene expression in abdominal subcutaneous adipose tissue in persons with the metabolic syndrome: the FUNGENUT Study. Am J Clin Nutr. 2007;85(5):1417-27.

[133] Allan CB, Lutz W. Life Without Bread; how a low-carb diet can save your life. 2000 McGraw-Hill. New York.

[134] DasUN. Essential fatty acids and their metabolites could function as endogenous HMG-CoA reductase and ACE enzyme inhibitors, anti-arrhythmic, anti-hypertensive, anti-atherosclerotic, anti-inflammatory, cytoprotective, and cardioprotective molecules. Lipids Health DIs. 2008;7:37.

[135] Levy E, Thibault L, Garofalo C, Messier M, Lepage G, Ronco N, Roy CC. Combined (n-3 and n-6) essential fatty deficiency is a potent modulator of plasma lipids, lipoprotein composition, and lipolytic enzymes. J Lipid Res. 1990; 31(11):2009-17.

[136] Damasceno NR, Pérez-Heras A, Serra M, Cofán M, Sala-Vila A, Salas-Salvadó J, Ros E. Crossover study of diets enriched with virgin olive oil, walnuts or almonds. Effects on lipids and other cardiovascular risk markers. Nutr Metab Cardiovasc Dis. 2011;21 Suppl 1:S14-20.

[137] Li SC, Liu YH, Liu JF, Chang WH, Chen CM, Chen CY. Almond consumption improved glycemic control and lipid profiles in patients with type 2 diabetes mellitus. Metabolism. 2011;60(4):474-9.

[138] Ros E, Núñez I, Pérez-Heras A, Serra M, Gilabert R, Casals E, Deulofeu R. A walnut diet improves endothelial function in hypercholesterolemic subjects: a randomized crossover trial. Circulation. 2004;109(13):1609-14.

[139] Wilson PW, Garrison RJ, Castelli WP et al. Prevalence of coronary heart disease in the Framingham Offspring Study: role of lipoprotein cholesterols. Am J Cardiol. 1980;46(4):649-54.

[140] Chester JG, Rudolph JL. Vital signs in older patients: age-related changes. J Am Med Dir Assoc. 2011;12(5):337-43.

[141] Cotugna N, Wolpert S. Sodium recommendations for special populations and the resulting implications. J Community Health. 2011;36(5):874-82.

[142] Sacks FM, Appel LJ, Moore TJ, Obarzanek E, Vollmer WM, Svetkey LP, Bray GA, Vogt TM, Cutler JA, Windhauser MM, Lin PH, Karanja N. A dietary approach to prevent hypertension: a review of the Dietary Approaches to Stop Hypertension (DASH) Study. Clin Cardiol. 1999;22(7 Suppl):III6-10.

[143] Moore R, Webb G. The K Factor: Reversing and Preventing High Blood Pressure Without Drugs. 1996 MacMillan Publ.

[144] Luther JM, Brown NJ. The renin-angiotensin-aldosterone system and glucose homeostasis. Trends Pharmacol Sci. 2011;32(12):734-9.

[145] Linnane AW, Kovalenko S, Gingold EB: The universality of bioenergetic disease: age associated cellular bioenergetic degradation and amelioration therapy. Ann NY Acad Sci, 1998; 854: 202-213.

[146] Folkers K, Langsjoen P, Willis R, Richardson P, Xia L-J, Ye C-Q, Tamagawa H: Lovastatin decreases coenzyme Q levels in humans. Proc Natl Acad Sci USA, 1990; 87: 8931-8934.

[147] Littaru GP, Ho L, Folkers K. Deficiency of coenzyme Q 10 in human heart disease. I. Int J Vitam Nutr Res. 1972;42(2):291-305.

[148] Gadaleta MN, Cormio A, Pesce V, Lezza AM, Cantatore P. Aging and mitochondria. Biochimie. 1998 Oct;80(10):863-70.

[149] Mortensen SA. Perspectives on Therpay of cardiovascular diseases with coenzyme Q10 (ubiquinone). Clin Investig. 1993;71(8 Suppl):S116-23.

[150] Hamilton SJ, Chew GT, Watts GF. Coenzyme Q10 improves endothelial dysfunction in statin-treated type 2 diabetic patients. Diabetes Care. 2009;32(5):810-2.

[151] Giovanni Ravaglia, Paola Forti, Fabiola Maioli, Luciana Bastagli, Andrea Facchini, Erminia Mariani, Lucia Savarino, Simonetta Sassi, Domenico Cucinotta, and Giorgio Lenaz Effect of micronutrient status on natural killer cell immune function in healthy free-living subjects aged ≥90 y. Am J Clin Nutr 2000;71:590–8

[152] Lockwood K., Moesgaard S., Yamamoto T., Folkers K. Progress on therapy of breast cancer with vitamin Q10 and the regression of metastases. Biochem Biophys Res Commun.1995 ;212(1):172-7.

[153] Lee JH, Jarreau T, Prasad A, Lavie C, O'Keefe J, Ventura H. Nutritional assessment in heart failure patients. Congest Heat Fail. 2011; 17(4):199-203

[154] Sole MJ, Jeejeebhoy KN. Conditioned nutritional requirements: therapeutic relevance to heart failure. Herz. 2002; 27(2):174-8.

[155] Keith ME, Walsh NA, Darling PB, Hanninen SA, Thirugnanam S, Leong-Poi H, Barr A, Sole MJ. B-vitamin deficiency in hospitalized patients with heart failure. J Am Diet Assoc. 2009;109(8):1406-10.

[156] Parcell S. Sulfur in human nutrition and applications in medicine. Altern Med Rev. 2002;7(1):22-44.

[157] Nagatomo Y, Tang WH. Intersections Between Microbiome and Heart Failure: Revisiting the Gut Hypothesis J Card Fail. 2015;21(12):973-80.

[158] Langsjoen H, Langsjoen P, Langsjoen P, Willis R, Folkers K. Usefulness of coenzyme Q10 in clinical cardiology: a long-term study. Mol Aspects Med. 1994;15 Suppl:s165-75.

[159] Shahzad K, Chokshi A, Schulze PC. Supplementation of glutamine and omega-3 polyunsaturated Fatty acids as a novel therapeutic intervention targeting metabolic dysfunction and exercise intolerance in patients with heart failure. Curr Clin Pharmacol. 2011;6(4):288-94.

[160] Loftus EV, Jr. Clinical epidemiology of inflammatory bowel disease: Incidence, prevalence, and environmental influences. Gastroenterology. 2004; 126:1504-17.

[161] Grassi M, Petraccia L, Mennuni G, Fontana M, Scarno A, Sabetta S, Fraioli A. Changes, functional disorders, and diseases in the gastrointestinal tract of elderly. Nutr Hosp. 2011;26(4):659-68.

[162] Talley NJ, Fleming KC, Evans JM, O'Keefe EA, Weaver AL, Zinsmeister AR, Melton LJ 3rd. Constipation in an elderly community: a study of prevalence and potential risk factors. Am J Gastroenterol. 1996;91(1):19-25.

[163] Kumar V, Sinha AK, Makkar HP, de Boeck G, Becker K. Dietary roles of non-starch polysachharides in human nutrition: a review. Crit Rev Food Sci Nutr. 2012;52(10):899-935.

[164] Musso G, Gambino R, Cassader M. Obesity, diabetes, and gut microbiota: the hygiene hypothesis expanded? Diabetes Care. 2010;33(10):2277-84.

[165] Nilsson AC, Östman EM, Knudsen KE, Holst JJ, Björck IM. A cereal-based evening meal rich in indigestible carbohydrates increases plasma butyrate the next morning. J Nutr. 2010;140(11):1932-6.

[166] Meijer BJ, Dieleman LA. Probiotics in the treatment of human inflammatory bowel diseases: update 2011. J Clin Gastroenterol. 2011;45 Suppl:S139-44.

[167] Abou-Donia MB, El-Masry EM, Abdel-Rahman AA, McLendon RE, Schiffman SS. Splenda alters gut microflora and increases intestinal p-glycoprotein and cytochrome p-450 in male rats. J Toxicol Environ Health A. 2008;71(21):1415-29.

[168] Purohit V, Bode JC, Bode C, Brenner DA, Choudhry MA, Hamilton F, Kang YJ, Keshavarzian A, Rao R, Sartor RB, Swanson C, Turner JR. Alcohol, intestinal bacterial growth, intestinal permeability to endotoxin, and medical consequences: summary of a symposium. Alcohol. 2008;42(5):349-61.

[169] Shindo K, Machida M, Fukumura M, Koide K, Yamazaki R. Omeprazole induces altered bile acid metabolism. Gut. 1998;42(2):266-71.

[170] Eom CS, Jeon CY, Lim JW, Cho EG, Park SM, Lee KS. Use of acid-suppressive drugs and risk of pneumonia: a systematic review and meta-analysis. CMAJ. 2011;183(3):310-9.

[171] Davis MA, Bynum JP, Sirovich BE. Association between apple consumption and physician visits: appealing the conventional wisdom that an apple a day keeps the doctor away. JAMA Intern Med. 2015;175(5):777-83.

[172] Del Piano M, Carmagnola S, Anderloni A, Andorno S, Ballarè M, Balzarini M, Montino F, Orsello M, Pagliarulo M, Sartori M, Tari R, Sforza F, Capurso L. The use of probiotics in healthy volunteers with evacuation disorders and hard stools: a double-blind, randomized, placebo-controlled study. J Clin Gastroenterol. 2010;44 Suppl 1:S30-4.

[173] I have no financial interest in this product or company.

[174] Judy Shabert, MD, MPH, RD Glutamine, The Ultimate Nutrient, 1994. Avery

[175] Moledina DG, Perazella MA. PPIs and kidney disease: from AIN to CKD. J Nephrol. 2016;29(5):611-6.

[176] Bradford GS, Taylor CT. Omeprazole and vitamin B12 deficiency. Ann Pharmacother. 1999;33(5):641-3.

[177] Mazziotti G, Canalis E, Giustina A. Drug-induced osteoporosis: mechanisms and clinical implications. Am J Med. 2010;123(10):877-84.

[178] Reimer C, Sondergaard B, Hilsted L, Bytzer P. Proton-pump inhibitor therapy induces acid-related symptoms in healthy volunteers after withdrawal of therapy.. Gastroenterology. 2009 Jul;137(1):80-7, 87.e1.

[179] Volta U, Bardella MT, Calabro A. Troncone R, Corazza GR. An Italian prospective multicenter survey on patients suspected of having non-celiac gluten sensitivity. BMC Med. 2014; 12:85.

[180] Xiao YL, Peng S. et al. Prevalence and symptom pattern of pathologic esophageal acid reflux in patients with functional dyspepsia based on the Rome III criteria. Am J Gastroenterol. 2010;105(12):2626-31.

[181] Stanghellini V, Frisoni C. Editorial: Reflux, dyspepsia, and Rome III (or Rome IV?). Am J Gastroenterol. 2010;105(12):2632-4.

[182] Dropping Acid; The Reflex Diet Cookbook and Cure. Jamie Koufman, MD and Jourdan Stern, MD. 2010

[183] Korzenik JR. Case closed? Diverticulitis: epidemiology and fiber. J Clin Gastroenterol. 2006;40 Suppl 3:S112-6.

[184] Commane DM, Arasaradnam RP, Mills S, Mathers JC, Bradburn M. Diet, ageing and genetic factors in the pathogenesis of diverticular disease. World J Gastroenterol. 2009;15(20):2479-88.

[185] Tarleton S, DiBaise JK. Low-residue diet in diverticular disease: putting an end to a myth. Nutr Clin Pract. 2011;26(2):137-42.

[186] Marcason W. What is the Latest Research Regarding the Avoidance of Nuts, Seeds, Corn and Popcorn in Diverticular Disease? J Am Diet Assoc. 2008; 108(11):1956 .

[187] http://www.surgeongeneral.gov/library/bonehealth/chapter_4.html #Prevalence

[188] Alarcón T, Gonzalez-Montalvo JI, Gotor P, Madero R, Otero A. A new hierarchical classification for prognosis of hip fracture after 2 years' follow-up. J Nutr Health Aging. 2011;15(10):919-23.

[189] JAMA, December 23/30, 1998—Vol 280, No. 24

[190] Nieves JW, Cosman F. Atypical subtrochanteric and femoral shaft fractures and possible association with bisphosphonates. Curr Osteoporos Rep. 2010;8(1):34-9.

[191] Cummings SR Nevitt MC, Browner WS et al. Risk factors for hip fracture in white women. Study of Osteoporotic Fractures Research Group. N Engl J Med. 1995;332(12):767-73.

192 Lin PH, Ginty F, Appel LJ et al. The DASH diet and sodium reduction improve markers of bone turnover and calcium metabolism in adults. J Nutr. 2003; 133(10):3130-6.

193 Food Surveys Research Group Dietary Data Brief No. 13. September 2014. Hoy MK, Goldman JD. https://www.ars.usda.gov/ARSUserFiles/80400530/pdf/DBrief/13_calcium_intake_0910.pdf

194 Kung AW, Luk KD, Chu LW, Chiu PK. Age-related osteoporosis in Chinese: an evaluation of the response of intestinal calcium absorption and calcitropic hormones to dietary calcium deprivation. Am J Clin Nutr. 1998;68(6):1291-7.

195 Xu. L. et al, Very low rates of hip fracture in Beijing, People's Republic of China ; The Beijing Osteoprosis Project. Am.J.Epedemiol. 1996 / 144 (9) / 901-907.

196 Xia WB, He SL, Xu L, Liu AM, Jiang Y, Li M, Wang O, Xing XP, Sun Y, Cummings SR. Rapidly increasing rates of hip fracture in Beijing, China. J Bone Miner Res. 2011. doi: 10.1002/jbmr.519.

197 Zalloua PA, Hsu YH, Terwedow H, Zang T, Wu D, Tang G, Li Z, Hong X, Azar ST, Wang B, Bouxsein ML, Brain J, Cummings SR, Rosen CJ, Xu X. Impact of seafood and fruit consumption on bone mineral density. Maturitas. 2007;56(1):1-11. Epub 2006 Jun 27.

198 Tilg H, Moschen AR, Kaser A, Pines A, Dotan I. Gut, inflammation and osteoporosis: basic and clinical concepts. Gut. 2008;57(5):684-94.

199 Fujita T, Fukase M. Comparison of osteoporosis and calcium intake between Japan and the United States. Proc Soc Exp Biol Med. 1992;200(2):149-52.

200 Tucker KL. Osteoporosis prevention and nutrition. Curr Osteoporos Rep. 2009 Dec;7(4):111-7.

201 http://www.health.harvard.edu/plate/healthy-eating-plate

202 http://www.choosemyplate.gov/index.html

203 Dietary Reference Intakes (DRIs): Recommended Dietary Allowances and Adequate Intakes, Vitamins; Food and Nutrition Board, Institute of Medicine, National Academies

204 Dietary Reference Intakes (DRIs): Recommended Dietary Allowances and Adequate Intakes, Elements. Food and Nutrition Board, Institute of Medicine, National Academies

205 Bolland MJ, Avenell A, Baron JA, Grey A, MacLennan GS, Gamble GD, Reid IR. Effect of calcium supplements on risk of myocardial infarction and cardiovascular events: meta-analysis. BMJ. 2010 ;341:c3691.

206 Reid IR, Bolland MJ, Sambrook PN, Grey A. Calcium supplementation: balancing the cardiovascular risks. Maturitas. 2011;69(4):289-95.

[207] Li K, Kaaks R, Linseisen J, Rohrmann S. Associations of dietary calcium intake and calcium supplementation with myocardial infarction and stroke risk and overall cardiovascular mortality in the Heidelberg cohort of the European Prospective Investigation into Cancer and Nutrition study (EPIC-Heidelberg). Heart. 2012;98(12):920-5

[208] Nieves JW, Barrett-Connor E, Siris ES, Zion M, Barlas S, Chen YT. Calcium and vitamin D intake influence bone mass, but not short-term fracture risk, in Caucasian postmenopausal women from the National Osteoporosis Risk Assessment (NORA) study. Osteoporos Int. 2008;19(5):673-9.

[209] Feskanich D, Willett WC, Stampfer MJ, Colditz GA. Milk, dietary calcium, and bone fractures in women: a 12-year prospective study. Am J Public Health. 1997;87(6):992-7.

[210] Rizzoli R, Stevenson JC et al. The role of dietary protein and vitamin D in maintaining musculoskeletal health in postmenopausal women: a consensus statement from the European Society for Clinical and Economic Aspects of Osteoporosis and Osteoarthritis (ESCEO). Maturitas. 2014.

[211] Delmi M, Rapin CH, Bengoa JM, Bonjour[c] JP, Vasey H, Delmas[d] PD. Dietary supplementation in elderly patients with fractured neck of the femur Volume 335, Issue 8696, Pages 1013–1016.

[212] White BL, Fisher WD, Laurin CA. Rate of mortality for elderly patients after fracture of the hip in the 1980's. The Journal of Bone and Joint Surgery. American Volume 1987, 69(9):1335-40.

[213] Clynes MA, Parsons C, Edwards MH et al. Further evidence of the developmental origins of osteoarthritis: results from the Hertfordshire Cohort Study. J Dev Orig Health Dis 2014;5(6):453-8.

[214] Lurati A, Laria A, Gatti A. et al. Different T cells' distribution and activation degree of Th17 CD4+ cells in peripheral blood in patients with osteoarthritis, rheumatoid arthritis, and healthy donors: preliminary results of the MAGENTA CLICAO study. Open Access Rheumatol. 2015 Oct 16;7:63-68.

[215] Alkan G, Akgol G. Do vitamin D levels affect the clinical prognosis of patients with knee osteoarthritis? J Back Musculoskelet Rehabil. 2016 Mar 27.

[216] Sköldstam L, Hagfors L, Johansson G. An experimental study of a Mediterranean diet intervention for patients with rheumatoid arthritis. Ann Rheum Dis. 2003;62(3):208-14.

[217] Zamani B, Golkar HR, Farshbaf S, et al. Clinical and metabolic response to probiotic supplementation in patients with rheumatoid arthritis: a randomized, double-blind, placebo-controlled trial. Int J Rheum Dis. 2016;19(9):869-79.

[218] Moghaddami M, James M, Proudman S, Cleland LG. Synovial fluid and plasma n3 long chain polyunsaturated fatty acids in patients with inflammatory arthritis. Prostaglandins Leukot Essent Fatty Acids. 2015 Jun;97:7-12

[219] Deutsch L. Evaluation of the effect of Neptune Krill Oil on chronic inflammation and arthritic symptoms. J Am Coll Nutr. 2007;26(1):39-48.

220 Dawczynski C, Hackermeier U, Viehweger M, Stange R, Springer M, Jahreis G. Incorporation of n-3 PUFA and γ-linolenic acid in blood lipids and red blood cell lipids together with their influence on disease activity in patients with chronic inflammatory arthritis—a randomized controlled human intervention trial. Lipids Health Dis. 2011;10:130.

221 Brown PM, Hutchison JD, Crockett JC. Absence of glutamine supplementation prevents differentiation of murine calvarial osteoblasts to a mineralizing phenotype. Calcif Tissue Int. 2011;89(6):472-82.

222 Shakibaei M, John T, et al. Suppression of NF-kappaB activation by curcumin leads to inhibition of expression of cyclo-oxygenase-2 and matrix metalloproteinase-9 in human articular chondrocytes: Implications for the treatment of osteoarthritis. Biochem Pharmacol. 2007;73(9):1434-45.

223 Mobasheri A, Henrotin Y, Biesalski HK Shakibaei M. Scientific evidence and rationale for the development of curcumin and resveratrol as nutraceutricals for joint health. Int J Mol Sci. 2012;13(4):4202-32.

224 Fitzgerald K. A case report of a 53-year-old female with rheumatoid arthritis and osteoporosis: focus on lab testing and CAM therapies. Altern Med Rev. 2011;16(3):250-62.

225 Schauss AG, Stenehjem J, Park J, Endres JR, Clewell A., Vitale C, Fini M. Effect of the novel low molecular weight hydrolyzed chicken sternal cartilage extract, BioCell Collagen, on improving osteoarthritis-related symptoms: a randomized, double-blind, placebo-controlled trial. J Agric Food Chem. 2012;60(16):4096-101.

226 Bagchi D, Misner B, Bagchi M, Kothari SC, et al. Effects of orally administered undenatured type II collagen against arthritic inflammatory diseases: a mechanistic exploration. Int J Clin Pharmacol Res. 2002;22(3-4):101-10.

227 Schwartz SR, Park J. Ingestion of BioCell Collagen(®), a novel hydrolyzed chicken sternal cartilage extract; enhanced blood microcirculation and reduced facial aging signs. Clin Interv Aging. 2012;7:267-73.

228 Xie Q, Shi R, Xu G, Cheng L et al. Effects of AR7 Joint Complex on arthralgia for patients with osteoarthritis: results of a three-month study in Shanghai, China. Nutr J. 2008;7:31.

229 Alipour B, Homayouni-Rad A, et al. Effects of Lactobacillus casei supplementation on disease activity and inflammatory cytokines in rheumatoid arthritis patients: a randomized double-blind clinical trial. Int J Rheum Dis. 2014; 17(5):519-27.

230 Tukmachi E, Jubb R, Dempsey E, Jones P. The effect of acupuncture on the symptoms of knee osteoarthritis—an open randomised controlled study. Acupunct Med. 2004;22(1):14-22.

231 Cao L, Zhang XL, Gao YS, Jiang Y. Needle acupuncture for osteoarthritis of the knee. A systematic review and updated meta-analysis. Saudi Med J. 2012;33(5):526-32.

232 Chen X, Spaeth RB, Freeman SG, Scarborough DM, Hashmi JA, Wey HY, Egorova N, Vangel M, Mao J, Wasan AD, Edwards RR, Gollub RL, Kong J. The modulation effect of longitudinal acupuncture on resting state functional connectivity in knee osteoarthritis patients. Mol Pain. 2015;11:67.

[233] Ribeiro RT, Afonso RA, Guarino MP, Macedo MP. Loss of postprandial insulin sensitization during aging. J Gerontol A Biol Sci Med Sci. 2008;63(6):560-5.

[234] Tilg H, Moschen AR. Inflammatory mechanisms in the regulation of insulin resistance. Mol Med. 2008;14(3-4):222-31.

[235] Eid HM, Haddad PS. The Antidiabetic Potential of Quercetin: Underlying Mechanisms. Curr Med Chem. 2017;24(4):355-364.

[236] Orchard TJ, Temprosa M, Barrett-Connor E, Fowler S, Goldberg R, Mather K, Marcovina S, Montez M, Ratner R, Saudek C, Sherif H, Watson K; The Diabetes Prevention Program Outcomes Study Research Group; prepared on behalf of the DPPOS Research Group Long-term effects of the Diabetes Prevention Program interventions on cardiovascular risk factors: a report from the DPP Outcomes Study. Diabet Med. 2012 Jul 19.

[237] Liese AD, Weis KE, Schulz M, Tooze JA. Food intake patterns associated with incident type 2 diabetes: the Insulin Resistance Atherosclerosis Study. Diabetes Care. 2009;32(2):263-8.

[238] Lim S, Won H, Kim Y, Jang M, Jyothi KR, Kim Y, Dandona P, Ha J, Kim SS. Antioxidant enzymes induced by repeated intake of excess energy in the form of high-fat, high-carbohydrate meals are not sufficient to block oxidative stress in healthy lean individuals. Br J Nutr. 2011;106(10):1544-51.

[239] Abete I, Goyenechea E, Zulet MA, Martínez JA. Obesity and metabolic syndrome: potential benefit from specific nutritional components. Nutr Metab Cardiovasc Dis. 2011;21 Suppl 2:B1-15.

[240] Tappy L, Lê KA, Tran C, Paquot N. Fructose and metabolic diseases: new findings, new questions. Nutrition 2010;26(11-12):1044-9

[241] Rayssiguier Y, Gueux E, Nowacki W, Rock E, Mazur A. High fructose consumption combined with low dietary magnesium intake may increase the incidence of the metabolic syndrome by inducing inflammation. Magnes Res. 2006; 19(4):237-43.

[242] Rosanoff A. Rising Ca:Mg intake ratio from food in USA Adults: a concern? Magnes Res. 2010;23(4):S181-93.

[243] Barbagallo M, Belvedere M, Dominguez LJ. Magnesium homeostasis and aging. Magnes Res. 2009;22(4):235-46.

[244] Williams AD, Almond J, Ahuja KD, Beard DC, Robertson IK, Ball MJ. Cardiovascular and metabolic effects of community based resistance training in an older population. J Sci Med Sport. 2011;14(4):331-7.

[245] Tomlinson JW, Finney J, Gay C, Hughes BA, Hughes SV, Stewart PM. Impaired glucose tolerance and insulin resistance are associated with increased adipose 11beta-hydroxysteroid dehydrogenase type 1 expression and elevated hepatic 5alpha-reductase activity. Diabetes. 2008;57(10):2652-60.

[246] Shearer GC, Savinova OV, Harris WS. Fish Oil –How does it reduce plasma triglycerides? Biochem Biophys Acta. 2012; 1921(5):843-51.

247 Ruggenenti P, Cattaneo D, Loriga G, Ledda F, Motterlini N, Gherardi G, Orisio S, Remuzzi G. Ameliorating hypertension and insulin resistance in subjects at increased cardiovascular risk: effects of acetyl-L-carnitine therapy. Hypertension. 2009;54(3):567-74.

248 Bugianesi E, Moscatiello S, Ciaravella MF, Marchesini G. Insulin resistance in nonalcoholic fatty liver disease. Curr Pharm Des. 2010 ;16(17):1941-51.

249 Ziyadeh N, McAfee AT, Koro C, Landon J, Arnold Chan K. The thiazolidinediones rosiglitazone and pioglitazone and the risk of coronary heart disease: a retrospective cohort study using a US health insurance database. Clin Ther. 2009 Nov;31(11):2665-77.

250 Mamtani R, Haynes K, Bilker WB, Vaughn DJ, Strom BL, Glanz K, Lewis JD. Association Between Longer Therapy With Thiazolidinediones and Risk of Bladder Cancer: A Cohort Study. J Natl Cancer Inst. 2012 Aug 9. [Epub ahead of print]

251 von Hurst PR, Stonehouse W, Coad J. Vitamin D supplementation reduces insulin resistance in South Asian women living in New Zealand who are insulin resistant and vitamin D deficient - a randomised, placebo-controlled trial. Br J Nutr. 2010;103(4):549-55.

252 Wang ZQ, Cefalu WT. Current concepts about chromium supplementation in type 2 diabetes and insulin resistance. Curr Diab Rep. 2010;10(2):145-51.

253 Racek J, Trefil L, Rajdl D, Mudrová V, Hunter D, Senft V. Influence of chromium-enriched yeast on blood glucose and insulin variables, blood lipids, and markers of oxidative stress in subjects with type 2 diabetes mellitus. Biol Trace Elem Res. 2006;109(3):215-30.

254 Saiyed ZM, Lugo JP. Impact of chromium dinicocysteinate supplementation on inflammation, oxidative stress, and insulin resistance in type 2 diabetic subjects: an exploratory analysis of a randomized, double-blind, placebo-controlled study. Food Nutr Res. 2016;60:31762.

255 Clandinin MT, Cheema S, Field CJ, Baracos VE. Dietary lipids influence insulin action. Ann N Y Acad Sci. 1993;683:151-63.

256 Wilmore DW. The effect of glutamine supplementation in patients following elective surgery and accidental injury. J Nutr. 2001;131(9 Suppl):2543S-9S; discussion 2550S-1S

257 Samocha-Bonet D, Wong O, Synnott EL, Piyaratna N, Douglas A, Gribble FM, Holst JJ, Chisholm DJ, Greenfield JR. Glutamine reduces postprandial glycemia and augments the glucagon-like peptide-1 response in type 2 diabetes patients. J Nutr. 2011;141(7):1233-8.

258 Menge BA, Schrader H, Ritter PR, Ellrichmann M, Uhl W, Schmidt WE, Meier JJ. Selective amino acid deficiency in patients with impaired glucose tolerance and type 2 diabetes. Regul Pept. 2010;160(1-3):75-80.

259 Krause MS, McClenaghan NH, Flatt PR, de Bittencourt PI, Murphy C, Newsholme P. L-arginine is essential for pancreatic β-cell functional integrity, metabolism and defense from inflammatory challenge. J Endocrinol. 2011;211(1):87-97.

260 Silva N, Atlantis E, Ismail K. A review of the association between depression and insulin resistance: pitfalls of secondary analyses or a promising new approach to prevention of type 2 diabetes? Curr Psychiatry Rep. 2012;14(1):8-14.

261 Stuart MJ, Baune BT. Depression and type 2 diabetes: inflammatory mechanisms of a psychoneuroendocrine co-morbidity. Neurosci Biobehav Rev. 2012;36(1):658-76.

262 Ajilore O, Haroon E, Kumaran S, Darwin C, Binesh N, Mintz J, Miller J, Thomas MA, Kumar A. Measurement of brain metabolites in patients with type 2 diabetes and major depression using proton magnetic resonance spectroscopy. Neuropsychopharmacology. 2007;32(6):1224-31.

263 Young LS, Bye R, Scheltinga M, Ziegler TR, Jacobs DO, Wilmore DW. Patients receiving glutamine-supplemented intravenous feedings report an improvement in mood. JPEN J Parenter Enteral Nutr. 1993;17(5):422-7.

264 Maggio M, Lauretani F, Ceda GP, Bandinelli S, Basaria S, Ble A, Egan J, Paolisso G, Najjar S, Jeffrey Metter E, Valenti G, Guralnik JM, Ferrucci L. Association between hormones and metabolic syndrome in older Italian men. J Am Geriatr Soc. 2006;54(12):1832-8.

265 Kintzel PE, Chase SL, Schultz LM, O'Rourke TJ. Increased risk of metabolic syndrome, diabetes mellitus, and cardiovascular disease in men receiving androgen deprivation therapy for prostate cancer. Pharmacotherapy. 2008;28(12):1511-22.

266 Atlantis E, Lange K, Martin S, Haren MT, Taylor A, O'Loughlin PD, Marshall V, Wittert GA. Testosterone and modifiable risk factors associated with diabetes in men. Maturitas. 2011;68(3):279-85.

267 Reynolds AC, Dorrian J, Liu PY, Van Dongen HP, Wittert GA, Harmer LJ, Banks S. Impact of five nights of sleep restriction on glucose metabolism, leptin and testosterone in young adult men. PLoS One. 2012;7(7):e41218. Epub 2012 Jul 23.

268 Arazi H, Damirchi A, Asadi A. Age-related hormonal adaptations, muscle circumference and strength development with 8weeks moderate intensity resistance training. Ann Endocrinol (Paris). 2013;74(1):30-5.

269 Smilios I, Pilianidis T, Karamouzis M, Parlavantzas A, Tokmakidis SP. Hormonal responses after a strength endurance resistance exercise protocol in young and elderly males. Int J Sports Med. 2007;28(5):401-6.

270 Vingren JL, Kraemer WJ et al. Testosterone physiology in resistance exercise and training: the up-stream regulatory elements. Sports Med. 2010;40(12):1037-53.

271 Morgantaler A. The Journal of Clinical Endocrinology & Metabolism , 2007 vol. 92 no. 2 416-417.

272 Rosano GM, Vitale C, Fini M. Testosterone in men with hypogonadism and high cardiovascular risk, Pros. Endocrine. 2015;50(2):320-5.

273 Yasui T, Matsui S, Tani A, Kunimi K, Yamamoto S, Irahara M. Androgen in postmenopausal women. J Med Invest. 2012;59(1-2):12-27.

274 Villareal DT, Holloszy JO. Effect of DHEA on abdominal fat and insulin action in elderly women and men: a randomized controlled trial. JAMA. 2004;292(18):2243-8.

275 Nair KS, Rizza RA, O'Brien P, Dhatariya K, Short KR, Nehra A, Vittone JL, Klee GG, Basu A, Basu R, Cobelli C, Toffolo G, Dalla Man C, Tindall DJ, Melton LJ 3rd, Smith GE, Khosla S, Jensen MD. DHEA in elderly women and DHEA or testosterone in elderly men. N Engl J Med. 2006;355(16):1647-59.

276 Lee NK, Sowa H, Hinoi E, Ferron M, Ahn JD, Confavreux C, Dacquin R, Mee PJ, McKee MD, Jung DY, Zhang Z, Kim JK, Mauvais-Jarvis F, Ducy P, Karsenty G. Endocrine regulation of energy metabolism by the skeleton. Cell. 2007 Aug 10;130(3):456-69.

277 Park K, Steffes M, Lee DH, Himes JH, Jacobs DR Jr. Association of inflammation with worsening HOMA-insulin resistance. Diabetologia. 2009;52(11):2337-44.

278 Morris MS, Sakakeeny L, Jacques PF, Picciano MF, Selhub J. J Nutr. 2010 Jan;140(1):103-10. doi: 10.3945/jn.109.114397. Epub 2009 Nov 11. Vitamin B-6 intake is inversely related to, and the requirement is affected by, inflammation status. J Nutr. 2010;140(1):103-10.

279 Ghashut RA, McMillan DC et al. Erythrocyte concentrations of B1, B2, B6 but not plasma C and E are reliable indicators of nutrition status in the presence of systemic inflammation. Clin Nutr ESPEN. 2017 Feb;17:54-62.

280 Zhang M, Gao Y et al. Association of serum 25-hydroxyvitamin D3 with adipokines and inflammatory marker in persons with prediabetes mellitus. Clin Chim Acta. 2017;468:152-158.

281 Farrokhian A, Bahmani F. et al. Selenium Supplementation Affects Insulin Resistance and Serum hs-CRP in Patients with Type 2 Diabetes and Coronary Heart Disease. Horm Metab Res. 2016;48(4):263-8.

282 Ylönen K, Alfthan G, Groop L, Saloranta C, Aro A, Virtanen SM. Dietary intakes and plasma concentrations of carotenoids and tocopherols in relation to glucose metabolism in subjects at high risk of type 2 diabetes: the Botnia Dietary Study. Am J Clin Nutr. 2003 ;77(6):1434-41.

283 Fang F, Kang Z, Wong C. Vitamin E tocotrienols improve insulin sensitivity through activating peroxisome proliferator-activated receptors. Mol Nutr Food Res. 2010;54(3):345-52.

284 Paolisso G, Balbi V, Volpe C, Varricchio G, Gambardella A, Saccomanno F, Ammendola S, Varricchio M, D'Onofrio F. Metabolic benefits deriving from chronic vitamin C supplementation in aged non-insulin dependent diabetics. J Am Coll Nutr. 1995;14(4):387-92.

285 Rizzo MR, Abbatecola AM, Barbieri M, Vietri MT, Cioffi M, Grella R, Molinari A, Forsey R, Powell J, Paolisso G. Evidence for anti-inflammatory effects of combined administration of vitamin E and C in older persons with impaired fasting glucose: impact on insulin action. J Am Coll Nutr. 2008;27(4):505-11.

286 Lautt WW, Ming Z, Legare DJ. Attenuation of age- and sucrose-induced insulin resistance and syndrome X by a synergistic antioxidant cocktail: the AMIS syndrome and HISS hypothesis. Can J Physiol Pharmacol. 2010;88(3):313-23.

287 Lautt WW, Macedo MP, Sadri P, Takayama S, Duarte Ramos F, Legare DJ. Hepatic parasympathetic (HISS) control of insulin sensitivity determined by feeding and fasting. Am J Physiol Gastrointest Liver Physiol. 2001;281(1):G29-36.

288 Mietus-Snyder ML, Shigenaga MK, Suh JH, Shenvi SV, Lal A, McHugh T, Olson D, Lilienstein J, Krauss RM, Gildengoren G, McCann JC, Ames BN. A nutrient-dense, high-fiber, fruit-based supplement bar increases HDL cholesterol, particularly large HDL, lowers homocysteine, and raises glutathione in a 2-wk trial. FASEB J. 2012;26(8):3515-27.

289 Ringseis R, Keller J, Eder K. Role of carnitine in the regulation of glucose homeostasis and insulin sensitivity: evidence from in vivo and in vitro studies with carnitine supplementation and carnitine deficiency. Eur J Nutr. 2012;51(1):1-18.

290 Golbidi S, Badran M, Laher I. Diabetes and alpha lipoic Acid. Front Pharmacol. 2011;2:69.

291 Padmalayam I. Targeting mitochondrial oxidative stress through lipoic Acid synthase: a novel strategy to manage diabetic cardiovascular disease. Cardiovasc Hematol Agents Med Chem. 2012;10(3):223-33.

292 Hamilton SJ, Chew GT, Watts GF. Coenzyme Q10 improves endothelial dysfunction in statin-treated type 2 diabetic patients. Diabetes Care. 2009 32(5):810-2.

293 Neal B, et al. Canagliflozin and Cardiovascular and Renal Events in Type 2 Diabetes. N Engl J Med. 2017;377(7):644-657.

294 Abete I, Goyenechea E, Zulet MA, Martínez JA. Obesity and metabolic syndrome: potential benefit from specific nutritional components. Nutr Metab Cardiovasc Dis. 2011;21 Suppl 2:B1-15.

295 Kim DJ, Xun P, Liu K, Loria C, Yokota K, Jacobs DR Jr, He K. Magnesium intake in relation to systemic inflammation, insulin resistance, and the incidence of diabetes. Diabetes Care. 2010;33(12):2604-10.

296 Das UN. A defect in the activity of Delta6 and Delta5 desaturases may be a factor in the initiation and progression of atherosclerosis. Prostaglandins Leukot Essent Fatty Acids. 200;76(5):251-68.

297 Horrobin DF. Essential fatty acids in the management of impaired nerve function in diabetes. Diabetes. 1997;46 Suppl 2:S90-3.

298 Han T, Bai JF, Liu W, Hu YM. A systemic review and Meta-analysis of α-lipoic acid in the treatment of diabetic peripheral neuropathy. Eur J Endocrinol. 2012 Jul 25.

299 Stracke H, Lindemann A, Federlin K. A benfotiamine-vitamin B combination in treatment of diabetic polyneuropathy. Exp Clin Endocrinol Diabetes. 1996;104(4):311-6.

300 Beli E, Clinthorne JF, Duriancik DM, Hwang I, Kim S, Gardner EM. Natural killer cell function is altered during the primary response of aged mice to influenza infection. Mech Ageing Dev. 2011;132(10):503-10.

301 Ravaglia, op cit in Co Q10 section Am J Clin Nutr. 2000 Feb;71(2):590-8. Effect of micronutrient status on natural killer cell immune function in healthy free-living subjects aged >/=90 y.

302 Vallejo AN, Hamel DL Jr, Mueller RG, Ives DG, Michel JJ, Boudreau RM, Newman AB. NK-like T cells and plasma cytokines, but not anti-viral serology, define immune fingerprints of resilience and mild disability in exceptional aging. PLoS One. 2011;6(10):e26558. Epub 2011

303 Song QH, Xu RM, Zhang QH et al. Glutamine supplementation and immune function during heavy load training. Int J Clin Pharmacol Ther. 2015;53(5):372-6.

304 Kaufman Y, Spring P Klimberg VS. Oral glutamine prevents DMBA-induced mammary carcinogenesis via upregulation of glutathione production. Nutrition 2008; 24(5):462-9.

305 Lull C, Wichens, HJ, Huub F, Savelkoul J. Antiinflammatory and Immunomodulating Properties of Fungal Metabolites. Mediators Inflamm 2005; 2005(2): 63–80.

306 Coffman RL. Origins of the TH1-TH2 model: a personal perspective. Nature Immunology 2006; 7(6): 539-541.

307 Haynes L, Linton PJ, Eaton SM, Tonkonogy SL, Swain SL. Interleukin 2, but not other common gamma chain-binding cytokines, can reverse the defect in generation of CD4 effector T cells from naive T cells of aged mice. J Exp Med. 1999;190(7):1013-24.

308 Yaqoob P, Calder PC. Glutamine requirement of proliferating T lymphocytes. Nutrition. 1997;13(7-8):646-51.

309 deJong N, Gibson RS, et al. Selenium and zinc status are suboptimal in a sample of older New Zealand women in a community-based study. J Nutr 2001; 131(10):2677-84.

310 Weksler ME. Immune senescence and adrenal steroids: immune dysregulation and the action of dehydroepiandrosterone (DHEA) in old animals. Eur J Clin Pharmacol. 1993;45 Suppl 1:S21-3; discussion S43-4.

311 Wintergerst ES, Maggini S, Hornig DH. Contribution of selected vitamins and trace elements to immune function. Ann Nutr Metab. 2007;51(4):301-23.

312 Inserra P, Zhang Z, Ardestani SK, Araghi-Niknam M, Liang B, Jiang S, Shaw D, Molitor M, Elliott K, Watson RR. Modulation of cytokine production by dehydroepiandrosterone (DHEA) plus melatonin (MLT) supplementation of old mice. Proc Soc Exp Biol Med. 1998;218(1):76-82.

313 Cannizzo ES, Clement CC, Sahu R et al. Oxidative stress, inflamm-aging and immunosenescence. J Proteomics 2011;74(11):2313-23.

314 Wu D, Meydani SN. Age-associated changes in immune function: impact of vitamin E intervention and the underlying mechanisms. Endocr Metab Immune Disord Drug Targets. 2014;14(4):283-9.

315 Simonsen L, Taylor RJ, Viboud C, Miller MA, Jackson LA. Mortality benefits of influenza vaccination in elderly people: an ongoing controversy. Lancet Infect Dis. 2007;7(10):658-66.

316 Janjua NZ1, Skowronski DM, Hottes TS, et al. Seasonal influenza vaccine and increased risk of pandemic A/H1N1-related illness: first detection of the association in British Columbia, Canada. Clin Infect Dis. 2010;51(9):1017-27.

[317] Thorlund K, Awad T, Boivin G, Thabane L. Systematic review of influenza resistance to the neuraminidase inhibitors. BMC Infect Dis. 2011;11:134.

[318] Venjatraman JT, Fernandes G. Exercise, immunity and aging. Aging (Milano). 1997;9(1-2):42-56.

[319] Shimizu K, Kimura F, Akimoto T, Akama T, Tanabe K, Nishijima T, Kuno S, Kono I. Effect of moderate exercise training on T-helper cell subpopulations in elderly people. Exerc Immunol Rev. 2008;14:24-37.

[320] Simpson RJ, Lowder TW, et al. Exercise and the aging immune system. Ageing Res Rev. 2012;11(3):404-20.

[321] Mimata Y, Kamataki A, Oikawa S, Murakami K, Uzuki M, Shimamura T, Sawai T. Interleukin-6 upregulates expression of ADAMTS-4 in fibroblast-like synoviocytes from patients with rheumatoid arthritis. Int J Rheum Dis. 2012;15(1):36-44.

[322] Bouguen G, Chevaux JB, Peyrin-Biroulet L. Recent advances in cytokines: therapeutic implications for inflammatory bowel diseases. World J Gastroenterol. 2011;17(5):547-56.

[323] Guerreiro CS, Ferreira P, Tavares L, Santos PM, Neves M, Brito M, Cravo M. Fatty acids, IL6, and TNFalpha polymorphisms: an example of nutrigenetics in Crohn's disease. Am J Gastroenterol. 2009;104(9):2241-9.

[324] Thomas S, Metzke D, Schmitz J, Dörffel Y, Baumgart DC. Anti-inflammatory effects of Saccharomyces boulardii mediated by myeloid dendritic cells from patients with Crohn's disease and ulcerative colitis. Am J Physiol Gastrointest Liver Physiol. 2011;301(6):G1083-92.

[325] Ignacio A, Fernandez MR, et al. Correlation between body mass index and faecal microbiota from children. Clin Microbiol Infect. 2016;22(3):258.e1-8.

[326] Fatouros IG, Chatzinikolaou A, Tournis S, Nikolaidis MG, Jamurtas AZ, Douroudos II, Papassotiriou I, Thomakos PM, Taxildaris K, Mastorakos G, Mitrakou A. Intensity of resistance exercise determines adipokine and resting energy expenditure responses in overweight elderly individuals. Diabetes Care. 2009;32(12):2161-7.

[327] Chad Waterbury. Huge In A Hurry: Get Bigger, Stronger, and Leaner in Record Time with the New Science of Strength Training. Rodale, Inc. 2008.

[328] Rodacki CL, Rodacki AL, Pereira G, Naliwaiko K, Coelho I, Pequito D, Fernandes LC. Fish-oil supplementation enhances the effects of strength training in elderly women. Am J Clin Nutr. 2012 Jan 4. [Epub ahead of print]

[329] Koopman R. Dietary protein and exercise training in ageing. Proc Nutr Soc. 2011;70(1):104-13.

[330] Melanson KJ, Summers A, Nguyen V, Brosnahan J, Lowndes J, Angelopoulos TJ, Rippe JM. Body composition, dietary composition, and components of metabolic syndrome in overweight and obese adults after a 12-week trial on dietary treatments focused on portion control, energy density, or glycemic index. Nutr J. 2012;11(1):57.

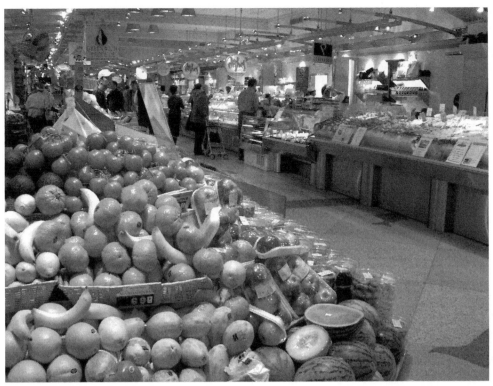

Photo by Karen Marlene Larsen

Made in the USA
Middletown, DE
22 August 2019